THE MAGIC HEALER'S DAUGHTER

KB TAYLOR

BOOT TOP BOOKS
Lacey, WA

The Magic Healer's Daughter is a work of nonfiction: letters, articles, family stories, and photographs from KB Taylor's collection.

Library of Congress Cataloging-in-Publication Data

Bishop, Karen (KB Taylor)

LCCN:2022948030

The Magic Healer's Daughter

KB Taylor-1" ed, Rev 3

p. cm: includes bibliographical references.

Summary: Based on the collections of KB Taylor

ISBN: 9798985655605

1. Magic Healers. 2. Mental Therapeutics. 3.) Sanipractic Physicians. 4. Mechano-Therapy 5. *Weltmerism*

Front Cover: Sarah Elizabeth (Lizzie) S.L. Snyder

Printed in the United States of America

March 2023

Boot Top Books

Lacey, WA

www.kb-taylor.com

AUTHOR'S NOTE

My great-grandmother Sarah Elizabeth (Lizzie) Snyder was a HEALER. After she passed away in 1936, her granddaughter, Viorene Gladys (née May) Muhlhauser, inherited her artifacts and later joined the Grays Harbor Genealogical Society. While growing up, young Gladys assisted in Lizzie's practice: handing out appointment cards, tending to the herbal garden, plus other tasks.

On my trips home to Washington State, my dad, sister and I would schedule an evening with Gladys. As we looked through her well-documented books, we'd listen to her stories. A treasured memory I hold dear.

By chance, I stopped at Gladys' home to visit her daughter. Gladys had passed away several months before. While there I noticed that her genealogy bookshelf had been replaced with stacked boxes. When I inquired, my cousin stated that she had tried to find a home for Gladys' artifacts, but to no avail and they were now slated for disposal. My husband was a very good sport when the twenty-plus heavy boxes arrived the next week on our doorstep.

Saving Lizzie's history bonded me to her even more. Plus, her first child, Mary Belle, was my great-grandmother, so it seemed fitting that I am the one telling Lizzie's story. I am grateful to be sharing her journey with you.

Author - KB Taylor

ACKNOWLEDGMENTS

A special thank you to Will Tollerton, Museum Coordinator of the Bushwhacker Museum, Nevada, Missouri. On his trips to the State Historical Society of Missouri annex in Kansas City, with my list in hand, he scoured through the artifacts. Thank you, Will. Your findings brought this book together.

To my husband, my sister, Diane, my cousin, Vickie, and to my Aunt Ruth. Thank you for your never-ending love and support and review of this book.

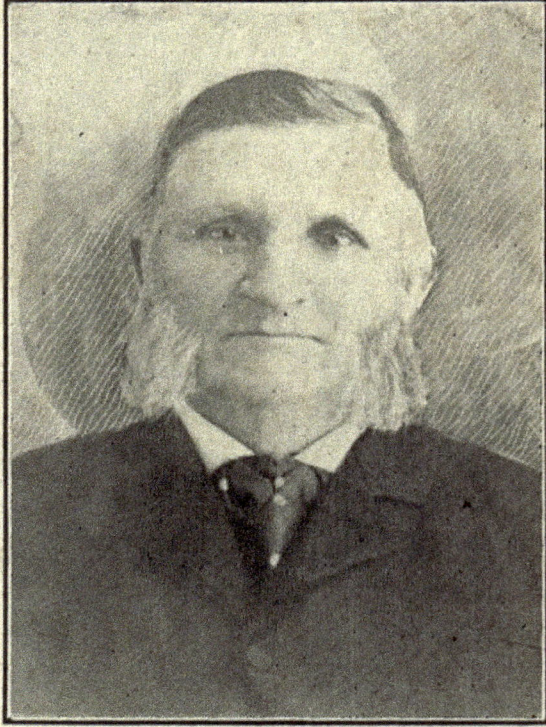

PROFESSOR W.B. WILSON
Magic Healer
(Author's collection)

INTRODUCTION

WHAT COULD THE reaction have been when W.B. Wilson at age sixty-three announced his news, Magnetic Healing? Once explained, was there shock and skepticism by what they were hearing? What did Lizzie think? It is known that she immediately stepped up to assist her father and accepted the challenge with the same enthusiasm that he possessed. But that would not have surprised those who knew her. She'd always been a risk-taker like her father, especially if it impacted people in a positive way.

It was surmised by family that this trait had been passed down by Lizzie's grandfather, Andrew Jackson Wilson. In addition to being a farmer, he had been a conductor on the underground railway in 1847, Oskaloosa, Iowa, fifteen years prior to the Civil War.[1]

In 1847 Lizzie's father, W.B. Wilson, was eleven and eldest of the children. Family records suggest that he aided his father in hiding the slaves. This had to have influenced his open mindedness to helping others by whatever means. Lizzie's actions with her healing and her friendship to Mr. Lee, a Chinese immigrant, proved in later years that she possessed similar views.

NOVEMBER 1900, LIZZIE'S father returned from Nevada,[a] Missouri as a Weltmer Institute graduate of magnetic healing. Magnetic healing was the method of curing diseases through the use of suggestions and hypnosis. It was referred to as the Weltmer Method, also known as Weltmerism. He had gone to the institute for treatment, but surprisingly returned as Professor W.B. Wilson, Magic Healer. With his course studies in hand and Lizzie at his side, he moved forward and created a successful practice in Aberdeen, Washington. Initially, it was an uphill battle to convince a lumber community filled with mill workers and loggers to accept this unorthodox trade, especially hypnosis.

Aberdeen, with so many seamen coming to the port on the lumber ships, was nicknamed one of the grittiest towns on the west coast.[2] But the majority of the permanent residents, including the businessmen along the wharfs, were upstanding, hardworking citizens. These were some of the people who Professor

---

[a] Nevada, pronounced *Naa-vey-da*.

Wilson sought as patients, but welcomed anyone in need. As Professor Wilson's healing practice grew, so did Lizzie's skills. She began reading his books, assisting with treatments, and enrolling in correspondence courses.

EARLY WOMEN MEDICAL practitioners were labeled as "wise women," healers, or midwives, but if the husband was a physician or ran an apothecary, the entire family assisted with mixing medicines, visiting the sick, and administering treatments.[3] Lizzie did the same for her father.

It was usually, the women who tended to the sick or dying neighbors. Nuns were also identified as medical practitioners with their convents turned into hospitals and portions of their gardens as medicinal herbal patches. Lay women healers were often vilified as dangerously incompetent because they lacked a classical education.[4] Lizzie later learned this firsthand; however, she pursued extra education. She went on to have a thriving healing practice of her own in the neighboring town of Hoquiam.

PACIFIC OCEAN

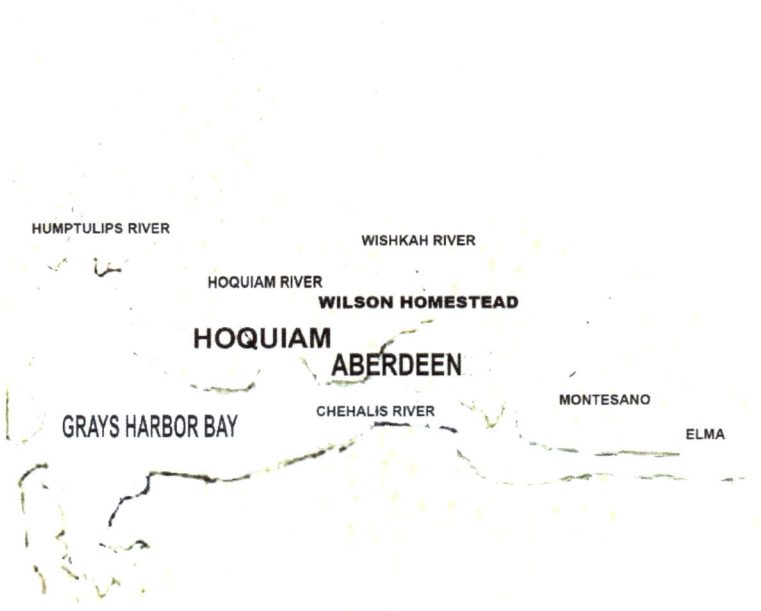

HUMPTULIPS RIVER

WISHKAH RIVER

HOQUIAM RIVER

WILSON HOMESTEAD

HOQUIAM

ABERDEEN

MONTESANO

GRAYS HARBOR BAY

CHEHALIS RIVER

ELMA

GRAYS HARBOR COUNTY, WASHINGTON STATE

CHEHALIS COUNTY RENAMED TO "GRAYS HARBOR COUNTY" IN 1915

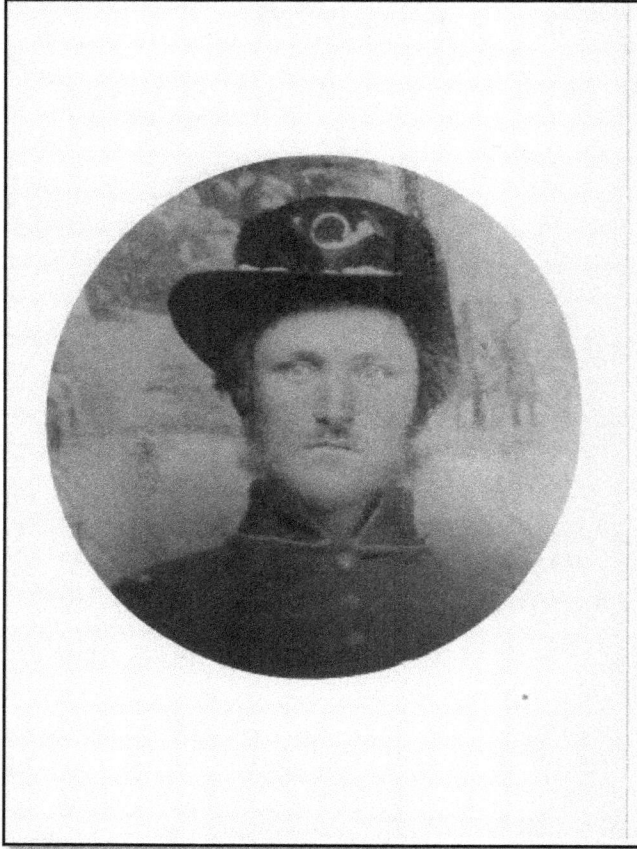

WILLIAM B. WILSON
28th Iowa Volunteer Infantry,
Union Army (1862-1865)
CIVIL WAR
(Author's collection)

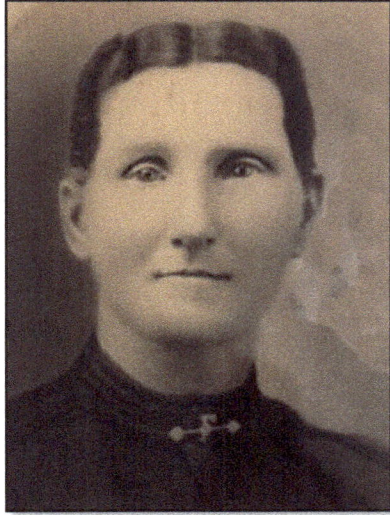

MARY WILSON (Mother)
(Author's collection)

William and Mary Wilson's Iowa/Missouri Children

Catherine	(1856, Iowa)
Andrew Jackson Jr. (A.J.)	(1859, Iowa)
Perry (1861 Iowa)	(1865, Iowa)
Sarah Elizabeth (Lizzie)	(1863, Iowa)
Leona (1865, Iowa)	(1870, Missouri)
Edward (1867, Iowa)	(1870, Missouri)
Wlm Jr. (1869, Iowa)	(1869, Iowa)
Charles	(1870, Missouri)

Oregon Territory Children

Lulu	(1872, Oregon)
Josephine	(1874, Oregon)
Alfred	(1876, Oregon)
Frank	(1879, Oregon)

1
THE EARLY YEARS

BORN BLIND on July 15, 1863, Hamburg, Iowa, Sarah Elizabeth (Lizzie) arrived after her father, William B. Wilson, had headed off to the Civil War. He learned of Lizzie's birth through a letter. When he returned home in late 1864, he was not the same man. Chronic colitis [b] had hospitalized him throughout the war with continued flare-ups. He also carried the scar of losing his eighteen-year-old brother, Albion, killed in battle.

In Iowa, the Wilson's had three more children, but also lost two. After the death of infant William Jr. in 1869, the family relocated to Holt, Missouri. It was in Missouri where Lizzie expanded her education. Her father had carved alphabet letters and numbers for her to count and spell out simple words like cat and dog. She often referred to these lessons as a blessing, because it meant that her mind could learn even though her eyes couldn't see.[1] The 1870 Missouri census records Lizzie attending school where she brought her alphabet carvings to class and sat with the younger students, listening as the teacher instructed.

As a blind child, she honed her memorization skills and was especially good at reciting stories. Holt, Missouri was the only location where the Wilson children received a classroom education. While living in Missouri, the Wilsons lost two more children. More hardship followed when William's health restricted him from working a full shift at the sawmill.

William's sister, Mattie, describes their life through a notarized affidavit later used for William's pension request for his time served in the Civil War. It was this condition that spearheaded his visit to the Weltmer Institute in Missouri for treatment thirty years later:

> *In the matter of the claim for the Pension of Wm. B. Wilson, C – 28 Iowa Infantry. Personally, came before me, a notary in and for said County and State, <u>Mattie A. McClure,</u> of the town of Pleasant Hill, County of Saline, State of Nebraska:*[2]

---

[b] Colitis—inflammation of the colon.

1

I have known claimant all my life, visited claimant and his family from date of discharge before and after I was married and lived by claimant. And my husband worked for claimant in a sawmill during the years of 1869 and 1870 at Corning, Holt County Missouri and saw him every day.

About six years ago he quit his trade and went into farming, not being physically able to follow his trade as head sawyer in the sawmill. Claimant's wages went from two dollars and fifty cents to three dollars per day while others doing the same work get from four to five dollars a day, on account of diarrhea as claimant was frequently laid off from work. (Pension of Wm. B. Wilson, C–28 Iowa Inf., Mattie A. McClure, 1888, 156.)

When Charles was born in October 1870, things looked up. He was healthy and strong. This was also the same year that eight-year-old Lizzie began seeing shadows. "Is that you I, see?" she asked her mother.[3] The next year, she traveled with her father to St. Louis for eye surgery. It is believed that she had a cataract-type surgery. One eye improved, the other remained blurred for the remainder of her life. Pictures reveal a lazy eye, causing the eye to wander inward and may have contributed to the blurriness. Shortly after her surgery, the family of six headed west for a new start and settled in Rainer, Oregon.

LIZZIE NOW NINE was learning to read and write. Between 1871 and 1879, she gained four siblings, but lost her eldest sister, Catherine, in marriage to Julio Xavier de Silva, a local businessman.

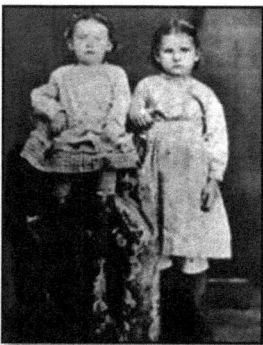

Lulu (2) and Lizzie (10)

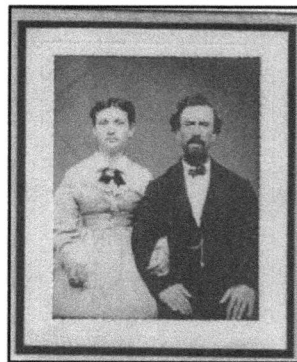

Catherine (16) and Julio Xavier de Silva (37)

In 1878, Lizzie now fourteen, was introduced to Emanuel Rodgers, Julio's first cousin. He was visiting from San Francisco.

Years prior, Emanuel and his father had sailed on a whaling ship from the Azores Islands, Portugal to America. At age twenty-four, he became a U.S. citizen.

With encouragement from Julio and her sister, Catherine, Lizzie and thirty-one-year-old Emanuel began courting. Two weeks following Lizzie's fifteenth birthday, they wed.

The next year, 1880, Mary Belle arrived. Lilly, was born two years later, 1882. Lilly's birth was overshadowed by Emanuel's failing health, later diagnosed as consumption. Shortly after, he died, leaving Lizzie a widow at barely nineteen.

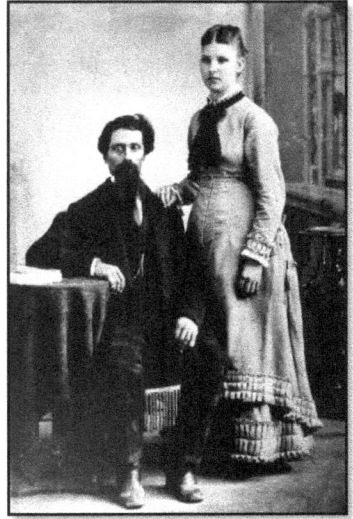

Emanuel and Lizzie Rodgers

THE PRIOR YEAR, Lizzie's parents had homesteaded to Washington State, three miles north of Aberdeen along the west bank of the Wishkah[c] River. Before settling there, Lizzie's father and her brothers, A.J. and Charles, cleared the land of trees, underbrush, and rocks. Luckily a portion had already been logged, leaving mostly scattered deep-rooted stumps. The Wishkah Valley was easily accessible by rowboat and one of the last settled areas, but among the first exploited for its remarkable timber.[4] With her mother's urging, Lizzie and her daughters boarded a steamboat north to Aberdeen.

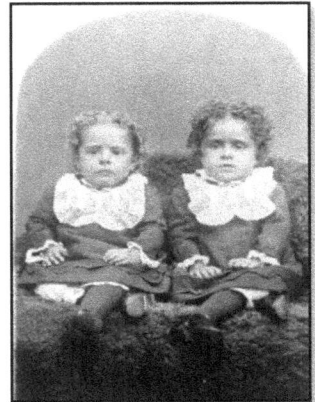

Lilly and Mary Belle Rodgers (1883)

LIZZIE HAD ONLY been widowed four months when her father brought forty-four-year-old Swedish laborer, William Hanson, to supper. The two worked at the Aberdeen shipyard. Little is known about Lizzie and Hanson's courtship, except for a Grand Ball program dated May 24, 1883 in Lizzie's belongings. The

---

[c] Wishkah (Wish-Kaah), a Native-American word meaning *stinking water*.

Grand Ball was sponsored by the Masonic Order, and more than likely, one of the largest community events of the year. Seven months later, William and Lizzie married.

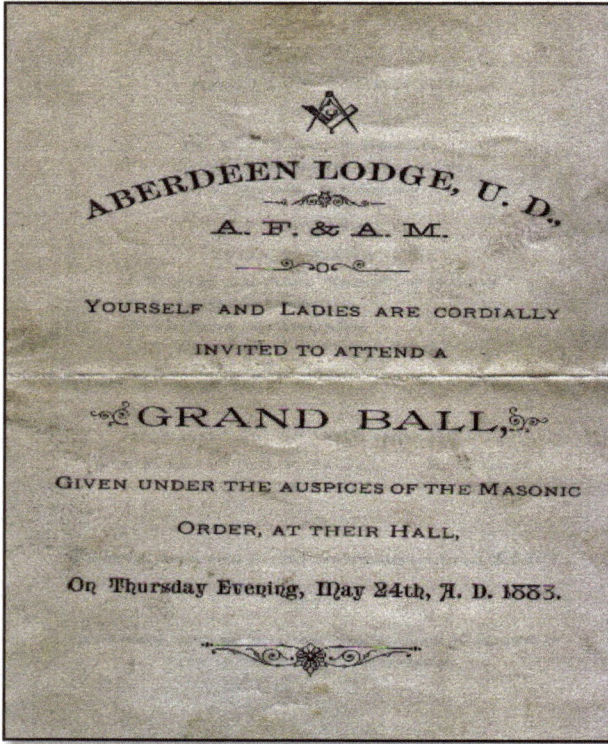

ABERDEEN LODGE, U. D.,
A. F. & A. M.

YOURSELF AND LADIES ARE CORDIALLY
INVITED TO ATTEND A

GRAND BALL,

GIVEN UNDER THE AUSPICES OF THE MASONIC
ORDER, AT THEIR HALL,

On Thursday Evening, May 24th, A. D. 1883.

1883 GRAND BALL PROGRAM
(Author's collection)

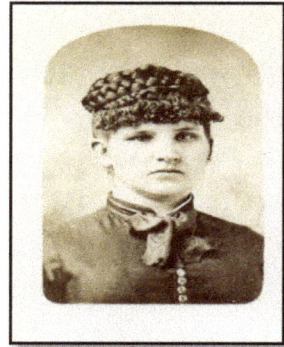

Lizzie (20)

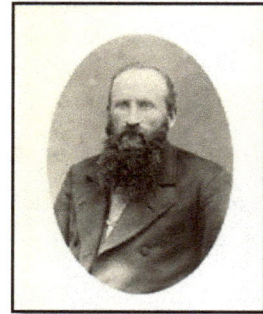

William Hanson (44)

Lizzie moved into the rooming house where William was living and her daughters remained with her parents. After William secured a better-paying position at the Hoquiam shipyard, they rented a small home near his job so that Lizzie's daughters could join them.

Little is known about their marriage during the early years, but it is known that when the honeymoon bloom wore off, his strong desire for the taste of liquor cropped up. It is believed that this was his prior lifestyle. When their first child, William Jr., arrived in late 1884, Lizzie was reeling from the death of her daughter, Lilly, who had died several months before. She prayed with the birth of a son, that William Sr. would change his ways, instead their marriage worsened.[5] In 1885, another son, Charles, arrived but he lived less than one year.

By 1888, Lizzie and William had been married four years and were expecting another child. Lizzie's state of mind is unknown, but her actions revealed undisputable courage. Three months before giving birth to son, Lester, she kicked William Hanson out of her life. Now age twenty-five, Lizzie had been widowed, divorced, buried two children, and had no source of income, but she had three children to raise: Mary Belle (8), William (4) and newborn, Lester.

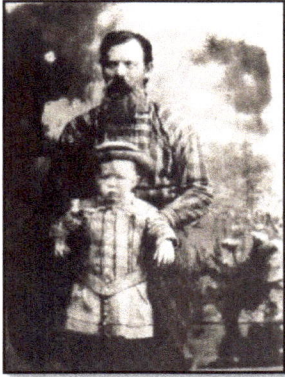

**William Hanson Sr.
with son Willie
(William Jr.)**

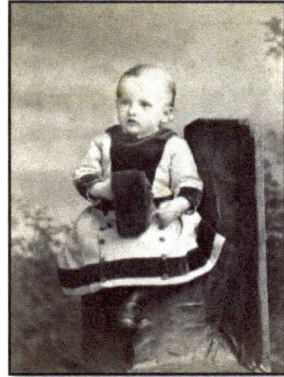

Lester

During the boy's teenage years, William Hanson Sr. reunited with his sons, but they never referred to him as father, instead addressed him as William Sr.

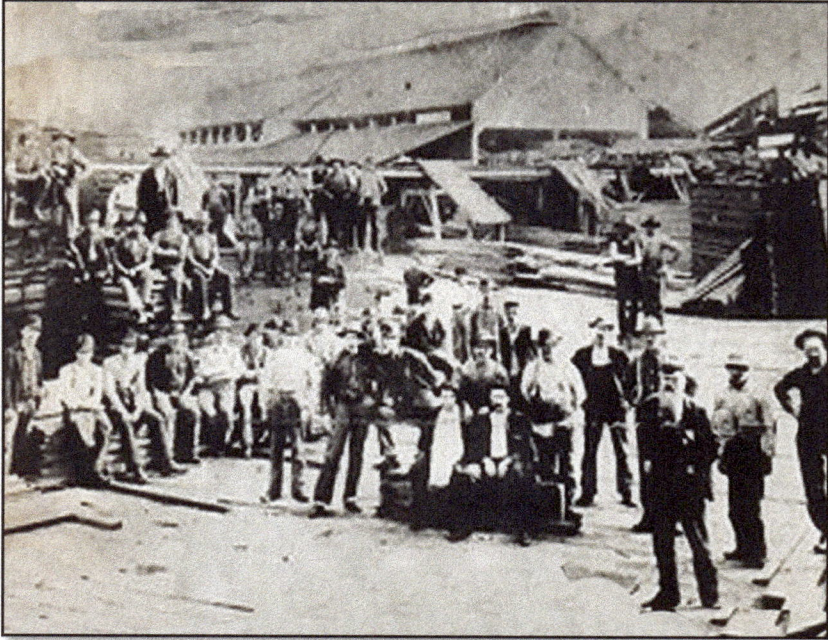

Northwestern Lumber Company
(Author's collection)

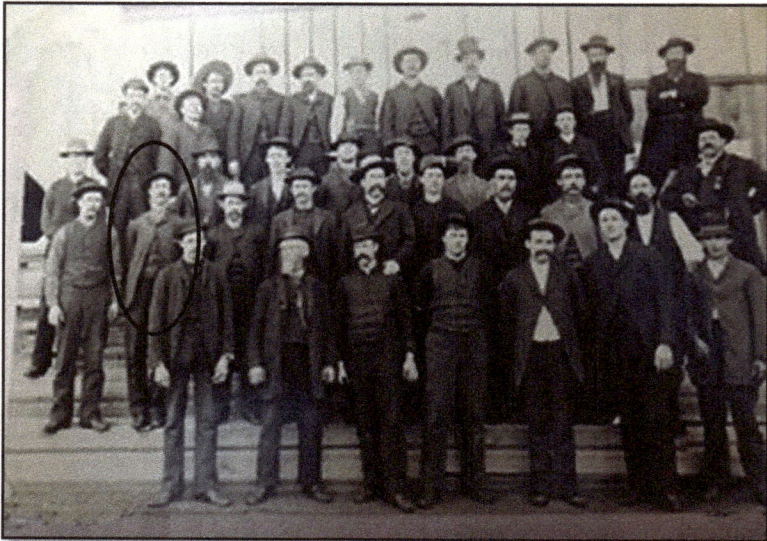

L to R (second row) John Snyder
Edger at Northwestern Lumber
(Author's collection)

2
BOARDINGHOUSE

IN 1888 WHEN THE CLASSIFIEDS advertised for a live-in cook and caretaker at a boardinghouse on the corner of 11th and J Street in Hoquiam, Lizzie applied. At least thirty men lived at the boardinghouse. The small rooms were shared by at least two in a double bed and more than likely had straw-filled mattresses with the local duck and goose feather downs for cushioning, plus a small table or dresser and a hook for clothes.

Most of the men worked at the Northwestern Lumber Company down the street and this boardinghouse may have been one of the establishments owned by the mill. Mill-owned boardinghouses usually lacked character—no large front porch, no sitting-room parlor or oversized windows. It was stated that some of the men would roll out of bed, saunter into the large dining room, and start dishing up. "More coffee," maybe some would say with a *please* or a *thank you.* Others may have been stragglers to the table, but when the mill whistle shrilled, they'd grab their lunch packs and take off in a full run.

What Lizzie didn't realize at the time, not many desired this job. The boardinghouse was in the older section of Hoquiam and considered a bit roughneck with all the nearby saloons. Up the block on 11th Street toward the river, were the "Ladies" of the restricted district. With strict Christian beliefs, Lizzie attended church weekly. It must have been a shock when she first saw the ladies in their long skirts hemmed with ruffles and flounces, held high showing their ankles. These ladies also wore long feather boas and wide plumed hats as they strolled up and down the planked walkways in front of their houses.

Sadly, she couldn't bring Mary Belle, now nine-years-old, into a boardinghouse with all men. Belle (Mary Belle) moved in with her grandparents at their Wishkah River home. She had been attending the more structured Hoquiam public school, but was transferred to the Wishkah one-room schoolhouse with her uncles, Frank and Fred Wilson.

Lizzie, William Jr. and newborn Lester settled into a large room on the top floor of the boardinghouse where they lived for the next eleven years (1888-1899). Lizzie's family wrote often with news about Mary Belle.

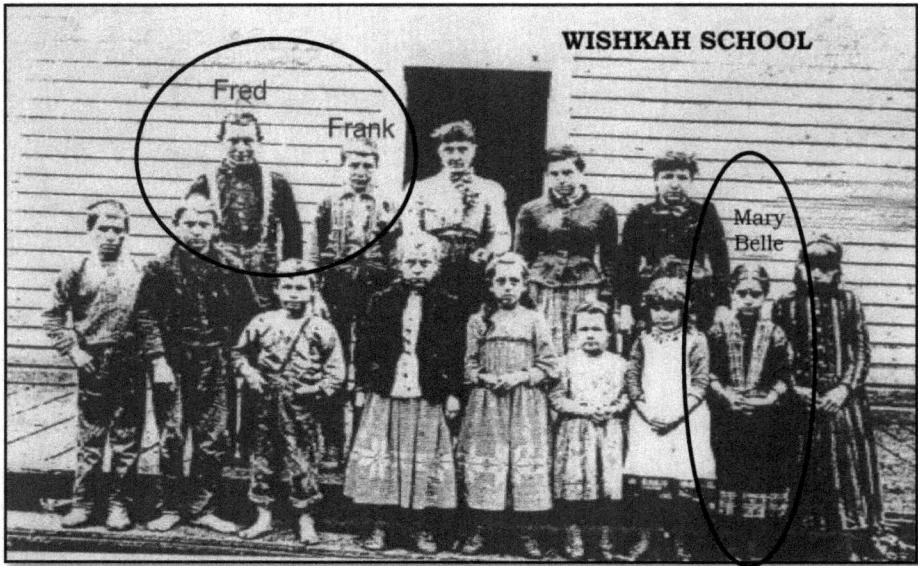

Mary Belle and Uncles Fred and Frank Wilson
Wishkah School 1889
(Author's collection)

Excerpt of Josie's 1893 letter:

> *Dear Sister Lizzie,*
> *Papa and the boys have been hauling in wood. Frank was sick Monday*
> *night; had a pain in both sides. Fred is cutting down a tree back of the*
> *barn this afternoon. School was out Friday. They had a meeting*
> *Saturday and are going to engage Mr. Achey to teach another term of*
> *four months. Mama is teaching Belle how to knit.* (Letter from Josie
> Wilson, Oct 4, 1893, 157-158.)

IT WAS IN 1889 at the boardinghouse where Lizzie met Mr. Lee. He was a Chinese immigrant and had been hired as the custodian in exchange for room and board. He and Lizzie became lifelong friends, but the Chinese people were not well received by all.

When the Chinese Exclusion Act of 1882 was passed by Congress, the Chinese remaining had to carry certificates of residence from the IRS. If caught without proper documentation, they faced hard labor and deportation. Bail was the only option, but had to be vouched by a white witness.[1] In 1890, the following incident occurred in Aberdeen, the neighboring town:

John Wing and his fellow pig-tailed country-men were ushered aboard the steamer "Wishkah Chief," transported to Montesano, and told to keep going.[2]

Some of the Chinese men came to work in the salmon canneries; others drifted to menial jobs and to gambling when not working. Then there were those who attached to the prostitution houses. There were no outcries when the Oriental population was shooed away.[3] (*The River Pioneers, Early Days on Grays Harbor* by Edwin Van Syckle, 379.)

The people of Hoquiam proved more tolerant, but Mr. Lee always ran his errands early to avoid any conflict.[4] He stayed close to the boardinghouse and to Lizzie. In addition to his duties, he also assisted Lizzie with the cleaning and the meals. Meals were included in the rent and served at specific times. More than likely, most breakfasts would have ham or bacon, eggs, toast, and homemade jams and jellies. Dinners had to be hearty too with meat, potatoes, and assorted side dishes, including a pie, tart or cake for dessert, which would have required frequent trips by Mr. Lee to the local butcher and grocers.

ON THE EVE OF the Panic of 1893, thirty-four-year-old John Snyder entered Lizzie's life. He was a new boarder and worked as an Edger, edging the ends of the boards, for the Northwestern Lumber Company, but had been well established in Hoquiam since 1889 as a member of the volunteer fire department.

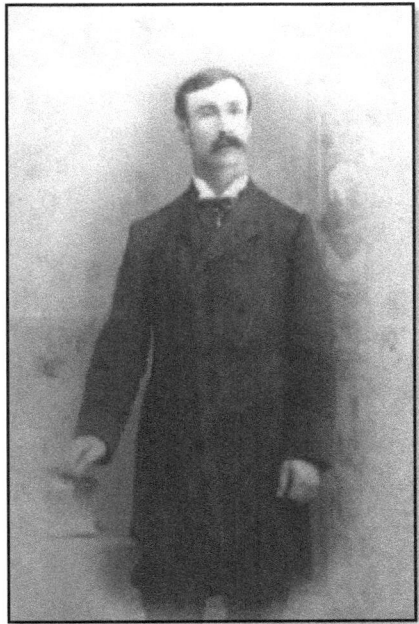

John Snyder
(Author's collection)

John and his brother, Wilber, left Colorado in 1887 and headed west in search of new opportunities. They settled in Hoquiam (Chehalis County, later renamed Grays Harbor County) and began buying cheap land. Letters from their aunt and uncle, farmers from Mitchellville, Iowa, paints a picture of what John and Wilber's life was like when they first arrived to the area. Excerpt September 22, 1889 letter:

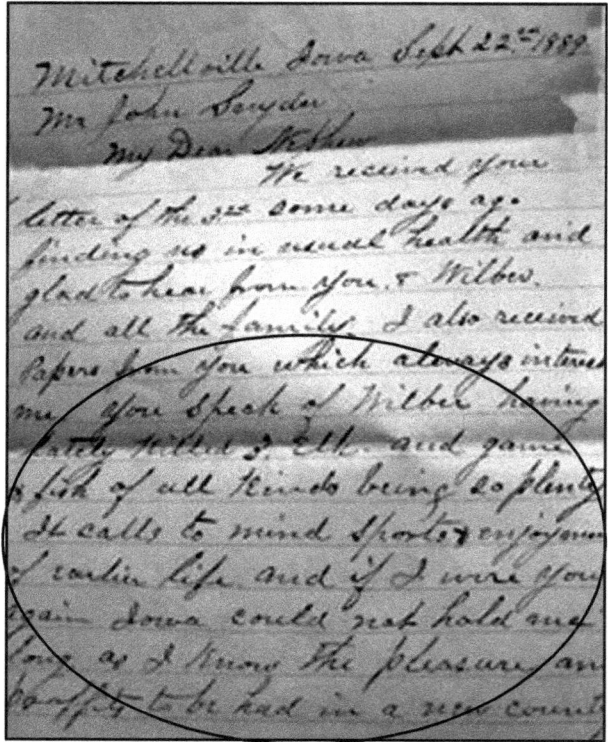

You speak of Wilber having lately killed an elk and game and fish of all kinds being so plenty. It calls to mind sports and enjoyment of earlier life. If I were young again, Iowa could not hold me long as I know the pleasure and proffits [sic] [d] to be had in a new country you speak of there, being good land to be taken in the unsurveyed [sic] district around that beautiful lake full of fish and abundance of game in the woods. (John Snyder's letter received from Mitchellville, Iowa, Sept. 22, 1889.) (Author's collection.)

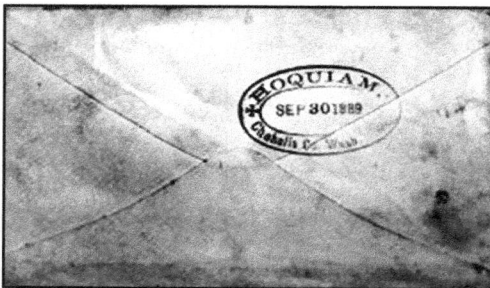

AS THE PANIC of 1893 swept the country, later causing a depression, Washington State was hit hard, especially the newer communities like Hoquiam and Aberdeen, heavily dependent on

---

[d] [sic], Latin: *sic erat scriptum* (thus was it written), quoted exactly as originally written.

logging. When the economy staggered, the Northwestern Lumber Company reduced staff. John Snyder was kept on half-time. The decline in boarders at the boardinghouse forced Lizzie into dressmaking. By the summer of 1894, she relocated to Tacoma and stayed with relatives while working in a textile factory. William Jr. and Lester remained at the boardinghouse under Mr. Lee's care.

Most factories were poorly ventilated, poorly lit, and kept the windows closed, forcing the workers to breathe in such contaminates as cotton lint and toxic fumes.[5] In addition to the miserable working conditions, the high speed of the sewing machines required close attention of the needle to avoid injury.[6]

Excerpt from John Snyder's July 1894 letter describes Lizzie's life during this period:

Hoquiam, Wash.
July 10, 1894

I am sorry that you have so poor place to work. The reason I didn't write real soon, I was waiting for payday to find out if I had enough money to spare to send you to come over, but I was disappointed. But next pay day look, and fare a firm [sic], if the mill does not shut down on the account of the Strike. I suppose there is excitable times in Tacoma. We can't get the mail half the time. But everybody is excited over the Strike. Your boys are well and everybody else. (J. Snyder letter to Lizzie in Tacoma, July 10, 1894, 159.)

The Panic of 1893 was partly due to the bankruptcy of the Philadelphia and Reading Railroad and to the passing of the "Sherman Silver Purchase Act," pushed by the Democrats after pressure by western mining interests. November 6, 1894, the midterm elections, the Democrats lost over 100 seats in the United States Congress. This was the largest single turnover in American history. Four senate seats were also overturned, giving the Republicans control of both houses. Democratic President Grover Cleveland, in his second term, was facing a catastrophic recession, a railroad strike, and massive demonstrations of jobless workers in Washington D.C. [7]

The depression lasted for four years, May 1893 through June 1897. Banks and businesses closed, railroads went bankrupt, credit froze, unemployment soared, and thousands lost their homes and savings. There were eighty-seven bank failures in Washington State, most due to depositors demanding to withdraw more than the banks had on hand.[8] In Hoquiam, five banks failed.[9]

While Lizzie was still working in Tacoma, John composed a letter, assessing her qualities. He wanted to give an honest viewpoint before asking her to marry him. One wonders if she provided the same type of critique of him? J. Snyder's 1894 letter:[10]

This is to certify that Mrs. was born in [sic] July 15, 1863, in the view of the moon sign was in burst, your nature is sympathetic, love of nature, of good ideas, of duty, a love of house and its surroundings. An ideal companion. Kind and affectionate to family, a good financer, care if no dictation amass [sic] a small fortune.

You have passed good opportunities by neglect. You are well provided with electricity. The gift of the power of authority in you is more than an average, well qualified to make all happy that is around you, your council is good and your decision is good and can be taken for granted.

You are sometimes superstitious, sometimes too much self, in company, you alienate attention and a good degree of modification, a word that you drop or utter has its firmness, you are the center of affection by your family, congenial nearby to your children's entreaties, a kind mother, good housekeeper--you may have had longing to become what you have tried and failed to become.

You have had experiences you could not understand, powers you were afraid to speak about, you wonder why the health you so sadly want is withheld from you, you may have longed and strived for earnestly for happiness and yet have failed to find it, you may have fought serious battles to overcome poverty and disaster, without a sign of success, it can be given to you the cause and cure of that state that makes poverty the initial step to the attainment of prosperity, it can be made plain to you and will uncover the highest and best within you,

you never have grasped the privilege that belongs to you. This power is implanted in you, a noble purpose. (J. Snyder letter to Lizzie in Tacoma, Nov, 1894, 160.)

The experiences she didn't understand were the loss of two children and two marriages, all faced by the age of twenty-five. Since childhood, she suffered from asthma and headaches from poor eyesight. Yes, she experienced poverty, but his positive statement of "how it would uncover the highest and best within you," and ending with "this power is implanted in you, a noble purpose," must have convinced her that he was the one. On December 23, 1894, she and John wed.

With vacancies at the boardinghouse, William Jr. and Lester moved into one of the empty bedrooms and Lizzie and John occupied the top floor. Mary Belle visited often, but continued living with her grandparents at the Wishkah until 1896 when Lizzie summoned her help. Lizzie was pregnant with daughter Jessie. Son, Lincoln, arrived the next year, 1897.

The year 1897 was also when major newspapers began printing stories about the Cuban people unfairly persecuted under Spanish rule. As a result, public sentiment was swayed against the Spaniards. The next year the Spanish-American War erupted in Cuba, several months after the sinking of the battleship, *Maine.*

Belle, now seventeen, was sensitive about her Portuguese complexion. She stopped going into stores, as many townspeople would give her odd stares, followed by whispers. To get away, she'd ride her bicycle out to Grays Harbor City—a rural community along the channel. It was there where she met Fred Cline.

Fred, twenty-three, was handsome, blond-haired, and a crew member on the tugboats. He also worked parttime as the light-tender, lighting the oil lamps along the channel and lived in a tent near the bay. Belle was known to be quite a talker, and he was a very shy man. When she announced to her mother that they were getting married, Lizzie was not pleased.

One can only imagine the conversation, especially after she discovered that they'd only known one another for a few weeks. Lizzie's two marriages at a young age had to have weighed heavily on her. She wanted a different path for her eldest daughter.

The newspaper article, published in the *Washingtonian* in 1897, offers insight to the situation: "The bride being but 17 years of age, her mother strongly objected to the marriage and refused to allow a license to be issued..."

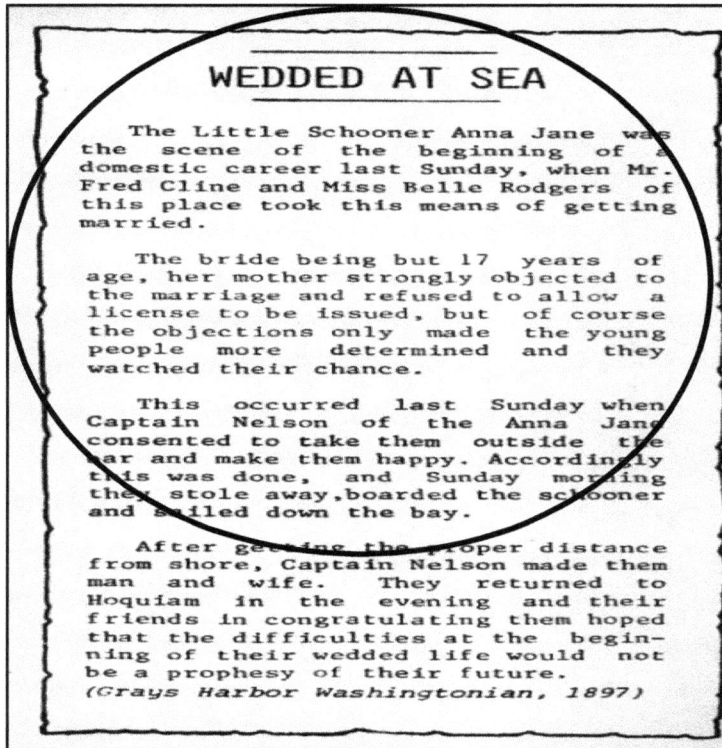

WEDDED AT SEA

The Little Schooner Anna Jane was the scene of the beginning of a domestic career last Sunday, when Mr. Fred Cline and Miss Belle Rodgers of this place took this means of getting married.

The bride being but 17 years of age, her mother strongly objected to the marriage and refused to allow a license to be issued, but of course the objections only made the young people more determined and they watched their chance.

This occurred last Sunday when Captain Nelson of the Anna Jane consented to take them outside the bar and make them happy. Accordingly this was done, and Sunday morning they stole away, boarded the schooner and sailed down the bay.

After getting the proper distance from shore, Captain Nelson made them man and wife. They returned to Hoquiam in the evening and their friends in congratulating them hoped that the difficulties at the beginning of their wedded life would not be a prophesy of their future.
(Grays Harbor Washingtonian, 1897)

(Author's collection)

Once Fred proved himself a hard worker, earning more than John was at the mill, Lizzie came to terms. Plus, the Spanish-American War had broken out and Belle and Fred living in a remote cabin along the Humptulips[e] River proved a wise choice.

Lizzie was also pregnant with her eighth and last child, Florence Effie Snyder. That same year, John purchased land on First Street in Hoquiam. With the help of Lizzie's father and brothers, they built a house. The family moved in the next year. William Jr., Lester, and Lincoln shared a bedroom as did Jessie and Florence. Living quarters with a separate entry were added to the back for

---

[e] Humptulips (Hum-tu-lups), Native-American word meaning *hard to pole*.

Mr. Lee. Mr. Lee later designed a healing garden in the backyard, which included bee boxes for honey. He lived the reminder of his life with Lizzie and John and was considered family. He is buried in the Snyder family plot.

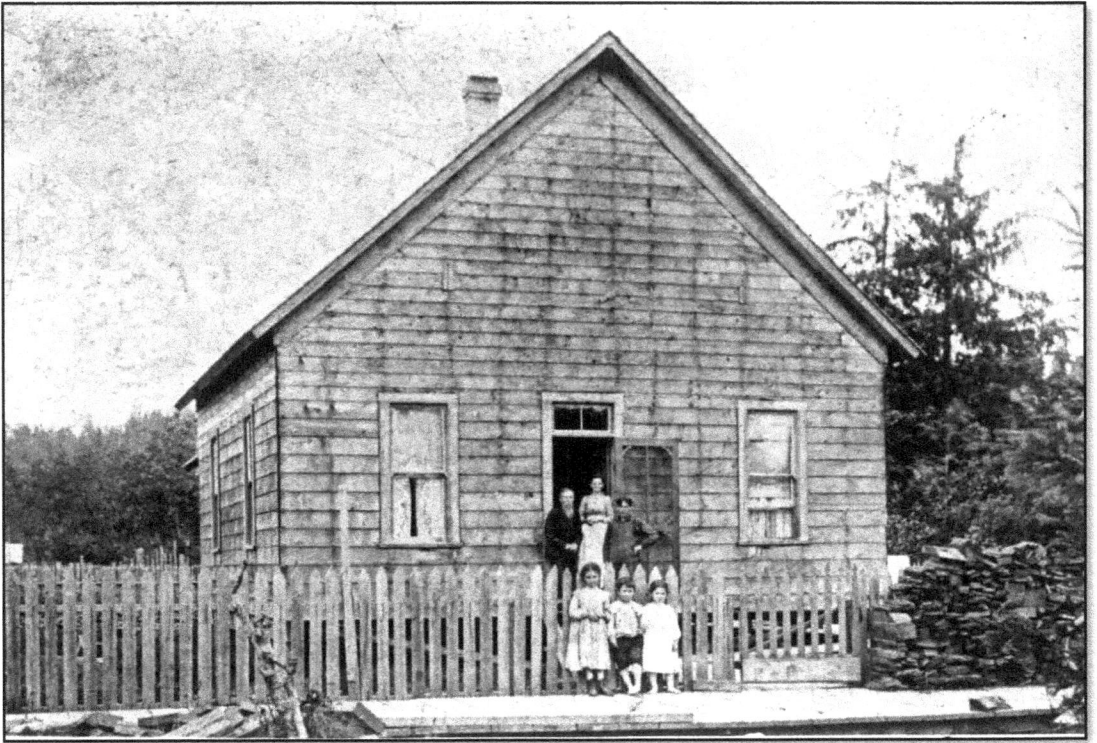

L to R (back)   Mr. Lee, Lizzie, and William Hanson Jr.
L to R (front) Jessie, Lincoln, and Florence Snyder

Snyder Family Home, First Street, Hoquiam, WA (1900)
(Author's collection)

Florence describes the Snyder family's early life on First Street, Hoquiam, WA. Excerpt from her 1962 letter to her daughter, Gladys:

My father was a [sic] edger man at the old Northwest Mill. He was very patriotic and took all us kids to political meeting [sic]. He was a councilman for Hoquiam. We always got in free at the circus. That is where Lincoln got butted by a goat.

15

Grandma Snyder ran a boarding house on 11th St. They moved to First St. when I was eleven months old. Only house on First St. at the time. Sawdust street at first then boards.

Playmates were frogs and log rolling. We was [sic] about a half block from the bay. No railroad there then but beautiful trees along where the railroad is now. It was a road where the track is now. We used to run through the empty houses & hotels at Grays Harbor City.

I was born on Eleventh St. (boardinghouse). Later on, Mother got pigs and Jessie, Lincoln & I went after the slop for them. We all took turns setting [sic] on the barrel. Someone in Hoquiam has a picture of all three of us on the cart. It was in a store window during Paul Bunyan Festival.

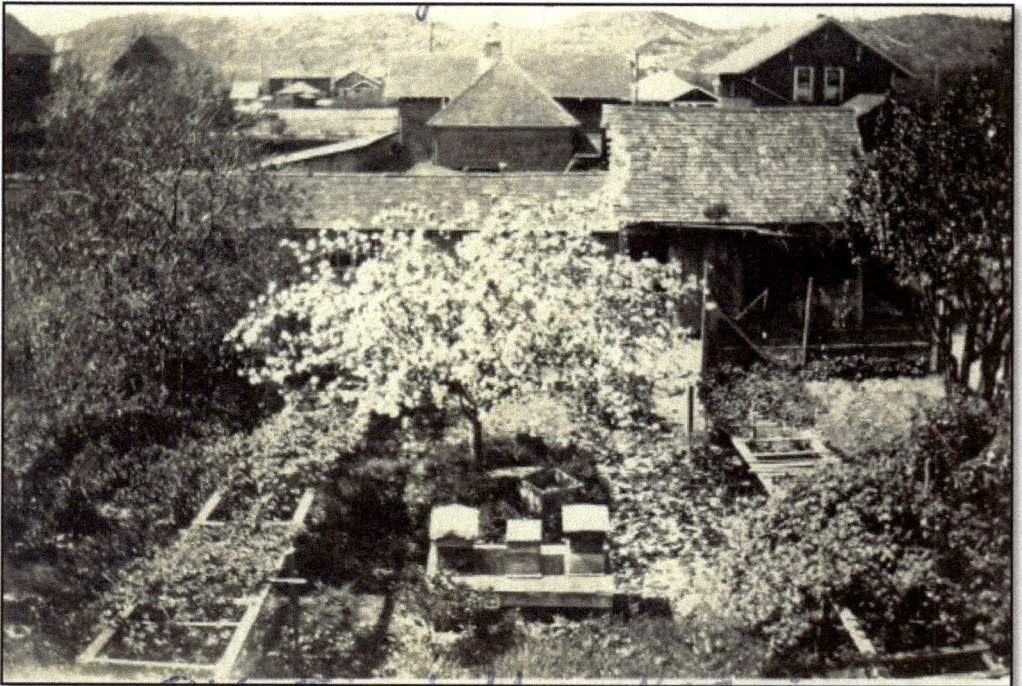

Lizzie's Backyard Healing Garden
Note the bee boxes for honey.
(Author's collection)

My father was a head man at the old Northwest Mill.

He was very political and took all us kids to political meetings.

He was a councilman for Hoquiam. We always got in free at the circus, that is where Lincoln got butted by a goat.

Grandma Snyder ran a boarding house on 11th St. They moved to ███ First St. when I was eleven months old. Only house on first st. at the time, Sawdust street at first then boards.

Playmates were frogs and log rolling. We was about a half block from the bay.

No railroad there then but beautiful trees along where the railroad is now. It was a road where the track is now.

We use to run through the empty houses & hotels at Grays Harbor City.

I was born on Eleventh St.

Later on Mother got pigs and June, Lincoln & I went after the slop for them. We all took turns setting on the barrel.

Some one in Hoquiam ha

a picture of all three of us on the cart It was in a store window during Paul Bunyon Festival.

Florence Oviatt

(Author's collection)

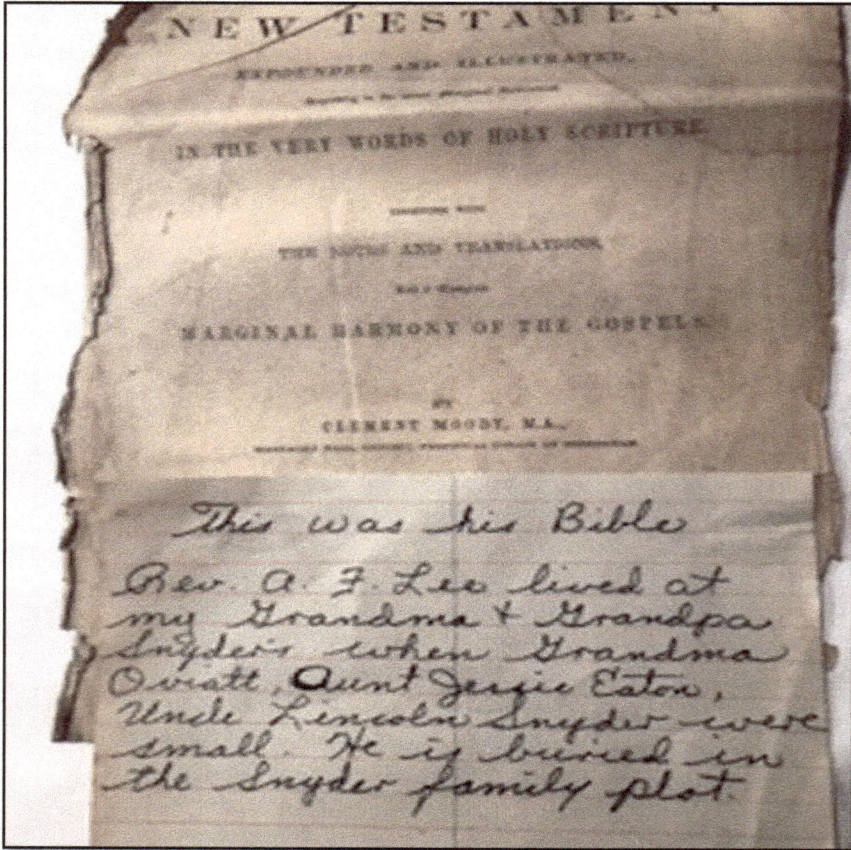

Page from Mr. Lee's Bible
Gladys Muhlhauser's Notation
(Florence Snyder's daughter)
(Author's collection)

3

WELTMER: The Healer

Children (12)
Catherine Wilson	B: 1856
Andrew Jackson Wilson	B: 1859
Perry H Wilson	B: 1861

William Burnsworth Wilson
B: 15 Jan 1836 in Indiana
D: 13 Jan 1910 in Montesano, Grays Harbor, Washington, United States

Mary Frances Howard Wilson
B: 22 May 1837 in Virginia, United States

Parents
Arthur Wilson
1810–1910

Arzilla
Johnson
1821–1872

William B Wilson
in the 1900 United States Federal Census

Detail | Source

Name:	William B Wilson
Age:	63
Birth Date:	Jan 1837
Birthplace:	Indiana, USA
Home in 1900:	Pleasant Hill, Saline, Nebraska
Sheet Number:	4
Number of Dwelling in Order of Visitation:	70
Family Number:	70
Race:	White
Gender:	Male
Relation to Head of House:	Brother in Law (Brother-in-law)
Marital Status:	Married
Marriage Year:	1856
Years Married:	44
Father's Birthplace:	Ohio, USA
Mother's Birthplace:	Ohio, USA
Occupation:	Carpenter
Months Not Employed:	9
Can Read:	Yes
Can Write:	Yes
Neighbors:	View others on page

Mary and William B. Wilson
(Author's collection)

Household Members	Age	Relationship
Mordecai Mcclure	63	Head
Martha A Mcclure	51	Wife
Merta Mcclure	24	Daughter
Arthur W Mcclure	17	Son
Hazel Mcclure	14	Daughter
Fredrick S Mcclure	9	Son
William B Wilson	63	**Brother in Law (Brother-in-law)**
Mary Wilson	64	Sister in Law (Sister-in-law)

1900 UNITED STATES FEDERAL CENSUS
William and Mary Wilson with William's sister, Martha A. (Mattie) McClure and
family, **PLEASANT HILL, NEBRASKA**
(Courtesy of NARA—National Archives and Records—public domain)

OCTOBER 1899, AN AD for the Weltmer Institute appeared in *The Seattle Post-Intelligencer.* Was it here where Lizzie's father first heard of Weltmer's healing school? Or was an ad seen by his sister, Mattie, who lived in Nebraska? Weltmer ads were flooding Midwest newspapers weekly and she could have easily read it in *The Kansas City Journal.* Regardless of how it was discovered, it prompted Lizzie's parents to make the cross-country journey to Nebraska, then on to Missouri.

Lizzie's father had suffered with chronic colitis for almost thirty-seven years, since the Civil War. It happened in 1863 when his troop had been shoved onto a cattle barge with several hundred others as they headed downriver to battle. The crowded conditions rendered many to the hospital.

Seeing the Weltmer ad must have given Lizzie's father hope of a cure or at least a lessening of the condition. The 1900 census shows her parents living with her father's sister, Mattie, in Pleasant Hill, Nebraska.

THE KANSAS CITY JOURNAL, JULY 1899
(Courtesy of the Library of Congress Digital Collection, Newspapers)
(Public domain)

MISSOURI-PACIFIC RAILWAY SCHEDULE
State Historical Society of Missouri (SHSMO) Artifact
(Courtesy of the Bushwhacker Museum, Nevada, Mo.)

From Nebraska, he caught the Missouri-Pacific train to Kansas City, and then to Nevada [f], Missouri. The entire trip from Mattie's Nebraska home to the Weltmer Institute would have taken approximately fifteen hours or so. Mary stayed behind in Nebraska with her in-laws.

---

[f] Nevada, pronounced *Naa-vey-da.*

THE WELTMER INSTITUTE was founded by Professor Sidney Abram Weltmer in February 1897, Nevada Missouri while he was on a circuit tour of southwest Missouri towns.[2] Years prior he had perfected his healing techniques to such success, he would find himself overwhelmed with patients. This very thing happened in Nevada, which led to his decision to make Nevada his permanent location.

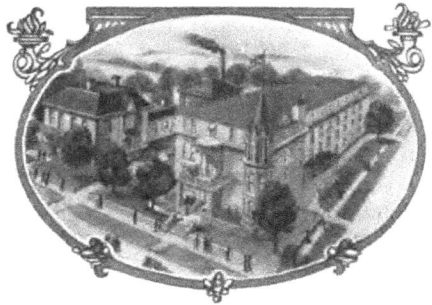

Weltmer Institute Drawing
(Author's collection)

Weltmer first operated out of a hotel and then relocated into a house. Two years later, he expanded into a seventeen-room mansion with a separate business building added next door.[3] His brother, John, and his eldest son, Ernest, soon joined him. His other sons, Tracy and Silas, later came aboard in administrative roles.[4] His two daughters stayed in the shadows with their mother.

To understand Weltmer's philosophy, one must understand the man. Born in Wooster, Ohio, 1858, Sidney Abram Weltmer was not educated by upper academic standards, but his mind and stamina were far beyond what a formal education would have provided. His father, however, attended the University of Pennsylvania and worked at Heidelberg University in Germany. His mother studied at Denison University and was the first woman to graduate from a collegiate course in the state of Ohio.[5]

Sidney attended public school and later borrowed medical books from a county doctor with hopes of becoming a doctor. Since childhood, he had suffered from weakness, which was later diagnosed as consumption, an ailment often fatal. Sidney refused to accept this death sentence and turned his studies to the Bible. At age nineteen, he became ordained and licensed as a Baptist minister. He put his faith in Christ's words, Mark 16:18:

> *And he said unto them go ye into all the world and preach the Gospel to every creature. He that believeth and is baptized shall be saved; but he that believeth not shall be damned. And these signs shall follow them that believe: In my name shall they cast out devils; they shall speak with new tongues. They shall take up serpents and if they drink any deadly thing, it shall not hurt them; <u>but they shall lay hands on the sick, and they shall recover.</u>*

He did recover, and in 1885, founded the Aikinsville Normal School, a private institution in Morgan County, Missouri, where he taught until 1889. In Sedalia, he established a public library and became a librarian for two years and also served as a professor at Robbins Business College. During this period, he expanded his studies and stated it all started at age seventeen when he came upon a book titled: *How to Become a Mesmerist.*[6] He went on to say, "that this little book, in connection with other articles from various works on the subject of what was then known as Animal Magnetism, excited a burning desire to know the phenomena connected with these subjects."[7] Sidney continued his studies with various authors on Mental Science as well as teachings of Jesus.

As a result, he began hypnotic experiments, which expanded into more studies and experiments. His conclusion was that the mind could control the body and that the effect of suggestion was a physical one brought about by the proper action of the mind. Resolved to test every manner of disease, he presented with one-hundred trials and reported success from the beginning.[8] His cases included: cancer, locomotor ataxia, tuberculosis, morphine habit, and malignant diseases. He also focused on Scripture Matthew 18:19: "If two of you agree on earth about anything you ask, then my Father who is in Heaven will do it for you."

AT THE WELTMER INSTITUTE, the student healer was taught to train his mind to concentration, to hold one thought to the exclusion of every other and hold it steadily, and if the patient shall be so instructed that he may become passive, an agreement in some degree would be reached, and a cure in some degree begun or established.[9] This philosophy was also used in absent treatment, where patients were sometimes hundreds or thousands of miles from their healer.

When a patient first met the healer, he was instructed to assume a passive attitude of mind. The healer seated the patient in a chair, explained that he was not going to be hypnotized, but had him close his eyes and think of a faraway pleasing object and to view it as a mental picture. The healer would then lay his hand upon the patient's head and, while watching the patient's eyelids and breathing, would put the relaxed patient in a state of sleep. The theory was that once the healer determined that the patient's mind was passive and receptive, the vibrations from the healer's mind would affect the patient's brain cells and allow the healer to begin his treatment. It was also important that the healer cultivate a positive attitude in the patient.[10]

THE DISCOVERY AND FORMULATION of the law of suggestion was credited to The Nancy School of Psychic Research. Their premise was: "When the conscious mind was in abeyance, the unconscious mind would do whatever you told it to do, believe whatever you said to it."

Weltmer followed this in his teachings, but did not agree that it was the whole of psychic healing as the Nancy School had affirmed. Weltmer asserted that the unconscious mind controlled all functions and activities of the physical organism (thoughts and ideas), and with the law of physical control and the law of suggestion, the healer could cause the patient's unconscious mind to heal its own body.[11] The concept of the unconscious mind had been known for years, but gained fame when Sigmund Freud's published work won him worldwide credit. Weltmer and his rival, Stanhope, had beaten Freud's theory by one year.[12]

The cardinal doctrine of Weltmerism was that two minds sounding as one responded to the same vibrations, and were synchronized and thinking the same thought. There could be no hypnotism unless two minds agreed; and when two minds, one being positive and the other receptive, agreed as to the thought of the positive mind, the passive mind may be said to be in a hypnotic condition.[13]

Laying on of hands was the physical sensation where suggestion entered the unconscious mind undoubted and unchallenged. For it to be most effective it was suggested to heat the hands. The process called "heating the hands" was achieved by various steps,[14] which included the raising and lowering of the arms and rubbing the hands briskly.

Weltmer also emphasized the importance of "Agreement." The Law of Being, the Creative force of the Universe, the Father in Heaven, God, was Law, and there was no way known to man by which this Law would act for man except through agreement. Jesus was the recognized author.[15] Absent Treatments followed the same Weltmerism principle, that the mind controlled the body through the exercise of the WILL, and the WILL, which brought the patient health or happiness or prosperity, was a compliance with the LAW.

Absent treatments, also referred to as home method of healing or home treatments, required prospective patients to complete a diagnostic questionnaire from the Weltmer Institute. Once reviewed by a Weltmer healer, treatment would be decided. In some cases, the healer would advise specific consultation with a surgeon, a physician, an osteopath or a chiropractor.[16] After the patient accepted the home-treatment plan, they were instructed on general hygiene and any specifics needed for them to reap the most benefit. Weekly, the patient was sent a report to update. After the healer reviewed their progress, he mailed back weekly suggestions. For the absent-treatment service, the patient paid a monthly charge of $5.00.

IN 1907, THE WELTMER Institute expanded the home treatment with the use of telepathy, conducting experiments over a period of years. The reports were studied, classified, and reported in Weltmer's Magazine. Telepathy was described as the co-operation of human intention with Infinite purpose. Each Thursday night during the experiment period, a telepathic message was sent from the institute, sometimes to as many as 8,000 receivers. One sender would broadcast to people in all parts of the world simultaneously. [17]

Professor Weltmer's treatment room was later turned into the Chapel of Silence. Various times during the day a Weltmer staff member would go into the Chapel where, conscious of the omnipresense—the presence of God everywhere at one time in which all minds were one—would think thoughts of health and strength for those whose names were recorded in that room. He'd harmonize his thought and the patients' thoughts with Divine purpose. This service was free to all who requested and could have their name added in the "Chapel of Silent Service" as long as they wanted. The only charge was for the weekly diagnosis portion of the home treatment.

In 1984, Dr. William S. Brink, executive director of the American Association of Professional Hypnotherapist, wrote the following about Sidney A. Weltmer: "What was being written seventy-five years ago is for the most part what is being written today. Today it just gets dressed up in high-tech jargon which makes it sound something altogether new." [18]

Author, Patrick Brophy, cofounder and curator of the Bushwhacker Museum at that time, concluded that Weltmer may have been ahead of his time. [19] A book published in 1910 titled: *Telepathy: Its Theory, Facts and Proof* by William Walker Atkinson, devoted three chapters to Weltmer's telepathic work and praised Sidney and Ernest Weltmer's frankness and fairness in their effort to prove or disprove the reality of extrasensory perception. [20] An excerpt from Chapter VIII: "The Weltmer Experiment will probably be followed by others along the same general lines. It is to be hoped that those who follow will remember to give full credit to the pioneer work performed in their behalf." [21]

THE WELTMER INSTITUTE had a substantial financial impact on the small town of Nevada. Railroads added additional cars to transport the thousands of patients who came to the institute for healing. Hundreds came to be trained in the Weltmer methods. The post office was upgraded to class one and a new building constructed to handle the massive volume.[22]

At its height, the institute treated 400 people a day and advised up to 150,000 persons a year by mail. It was reported that Weltmer employees carried bushel baskets of cash to the bank.[23] The institute employed 17 healers and over 100 stenographers and typists to process all of the correspondence. Weltmer also advertised in newspapers. Some of the ads provided information on speaking engagements, others described the healing with testimonials of those who were healed, and then there were ads offering course studies with an estimated salary that a Weltmer professor could earn: "Agents — learn a profession in 10 days that will net you $25 [g] a day the rest of your life."

He also created his own publishing company in 1898. One of his first publications was the *Magnetic Journal* and later renamed the *Weltmer Journal*. *Weltmerism* magazine ran in conjunction with the journal, but its magazine layout of supplementary photos accompanied by short editorials provided a polished view. Both publications showcased testimonials from patients with successful results where modern medicine had failed, and information about the school courses, lodging, and other relevant facts. More importantly, both served as advertising tools for the institute. The *Magnetic Journal* stopped publication in 1904 and reissued as *Weltmer Journal* intermittently through 1906 when it was then consolidated into *Weltmer's Magazine*.

---

[g] About $900 in today's money.

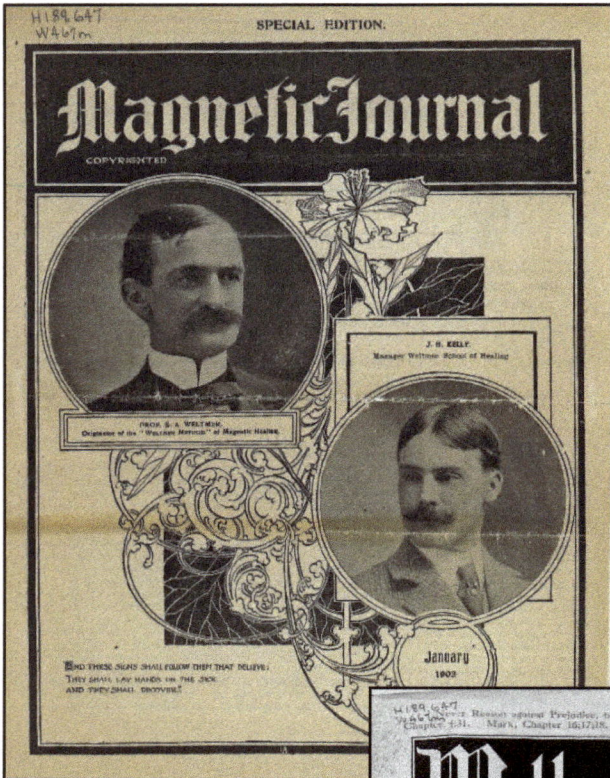

MAGNETIC JOURNAL
(1898-1904)
State Historical Society of
Missouri
(SHSMO) Artifact
(Courtesy of the Bushwhacker
Museum, Nevada, Mo.)

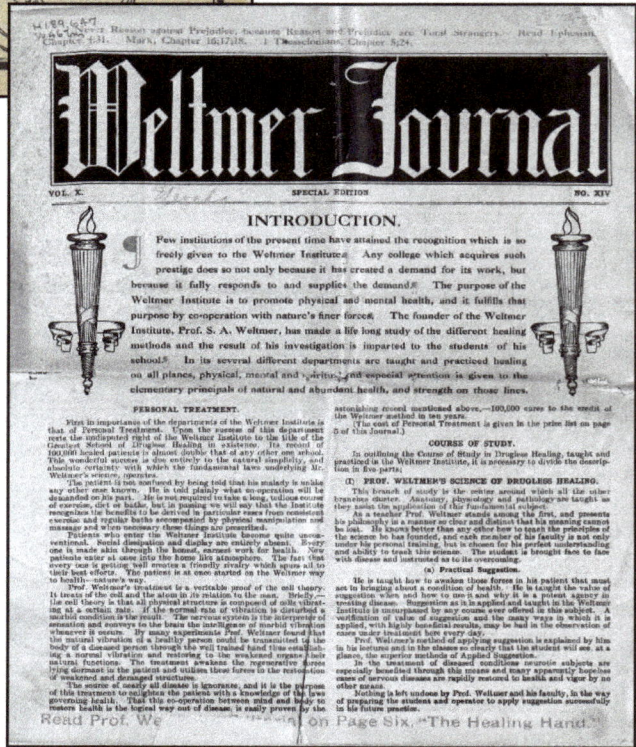

WELTMER JOURNAL
(1904-1906)
State Historical Society of
Missouri
(SHSMO) Artifact
(Courtesy of the Bushwhacker
Museum, Nevada, Mo.)

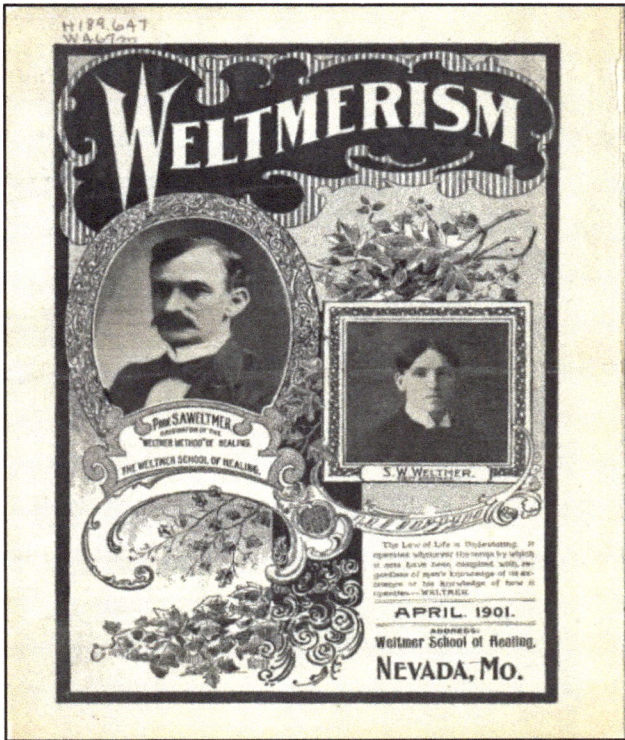

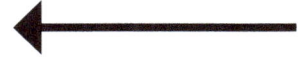

WELTMER'S MAGAZINE entered the scene in January 1901 as a monthly publication for ten cents a copy or a yearly subscription for a dollar. In addition to advertisements, Professor Weltmer and his sons and other credentialed spiritual leaders provided sermon-like editorials on various subjects, such as Weltmerism, psychic healing, and spiritual philosophy. It was also during this period that the "New Thought" movement was gaining steam and became a key component of the magazine.

New Thought was a mind-healing movement that originated in the United States in the late 1800's. Its origins were based on the teachings of Phineas Quimby (1802-1866), an American mesmerist and healer. Quimby used hypnosis as a means to healing, but also discovered he could heal by suggestion. He became convinced that disease was an error of the mind and not a real thing.[24] The Christian Science founder, Mary Baker Eddy, was a patient of Quimby's and shared in some of his views, but because of her faith, Christian Science deviated from his teachings. New Thought emerged through other religious avenues such as Unity Church and Church of Divine Science. Ralph Waldo Emerson, an American essayist, philosopher, and mentor to Henry David Thoreau, led the transcendentalist movement, which was also adopted by some into the New Thought theory.

New Thought philosophy embraces that God is omnipotent, omnipresent, and omniscient; and God is in all and all is in God. Its core principles and beliefs state: [25]

- Infinite Intelligence or God is everywhere,
- Spirit is the totality of real things,
- True human selfhood is divine,
- Divine thought is a force for good,
- Sickness originates in the mind,
- Right thinking has a healing effect.

And that "a higher power pervades all existence, and that individuals create their own reality via affirmations, meditation, and prayer."[26]

An affirmative prayer is a metaphysical technique that focuses on a positive outcome instead of a negative and affirms that the desired intention has already happened, rather than asking God to eliminate it.[27]

Not all of these principles aligned to Weltmer's. He believed that the power was all in the Creator. That the Creator in action was Law, and referred to the Creator by various names: Law, Law of Nature, Law of Being, God, and designated by Jesus Christ as "My Father which is in Heaven."

According to Weltmer, man's power did not consist in any inherent, inborn, latent ability that he possessed; his power

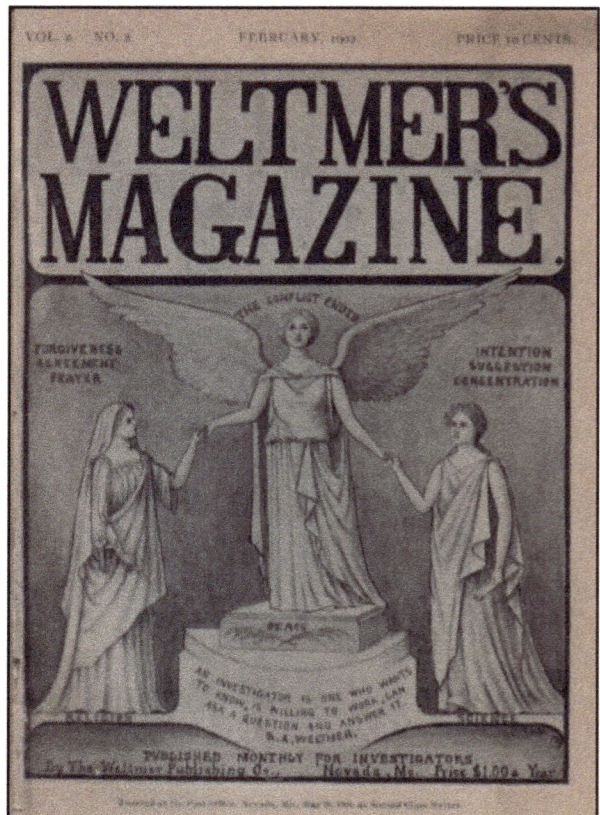

WELTMER'S MAGAZINE
(1901-1930)
State Historical Society of Missouri. Artifact
(Courtesy of the Bushwhacker Museum, Nevada, Mo.)

consisted solely in his ability to grasp the meaning of the Law that governed him and to comply with it. [28]

To expand the magazine's readership, Weltmer realigned his thinking, not in agreement to the New Thought movement, but to recognize their right to their beliefs by stating "honest convictions, founded upon reason, and respectfully expressed, would be welcomed for submission and publication." The March 1901 edition proclaimed itself devoted to spiritual philosophy, psychic healing, and the New Thought of present day. [29] In September 1905, the Fifth Annual Convention of the New Thought Federation was held at the Weltmer Institute.

AUGUST 1906, *Fulfillment*, a monthly metaphysical magazine, consolidated with *Weltmer's Magazine*. Its editor Grace M. Brown, an American writer and spiritual leader, who was instrumental in the New Thought movement, joined the Weltmer editorial staff. Her "Fulfillment" editorials and "Cozy Chats" were featured in *Weltmer's Magazine*.

WELTMER'S MAGAZINE
1907
State Historical Society of Missouri
(SHSMO) Artifact
(Courtesy of the Bushwhacker
Museum, Nevada, Mo.)

**Reference articles by Grace
M. Brown (circled)**

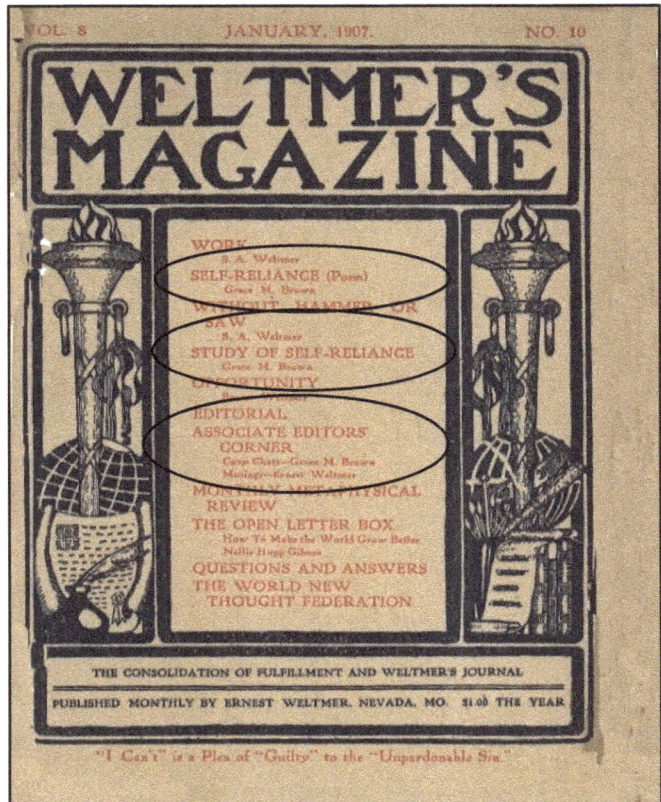

Note: consolidation of
Fulfillment magazine and
Weltmer's Journal.

Excerpt from Robert L. Stone's, Jr. paper, "Weltmer: Pioneer of Psychotherapy:"

Weltmer was noted for his generosity, hospitality, and public spirit. He amassed no fortune and spent his money as quickly as he earned it. He recognized the need for medical care and advocated the use of surgery if needed. He never assumed that he could cure everyone and never claimed to have miraculous powers.[30] (Bushwhacker Museum archives.)

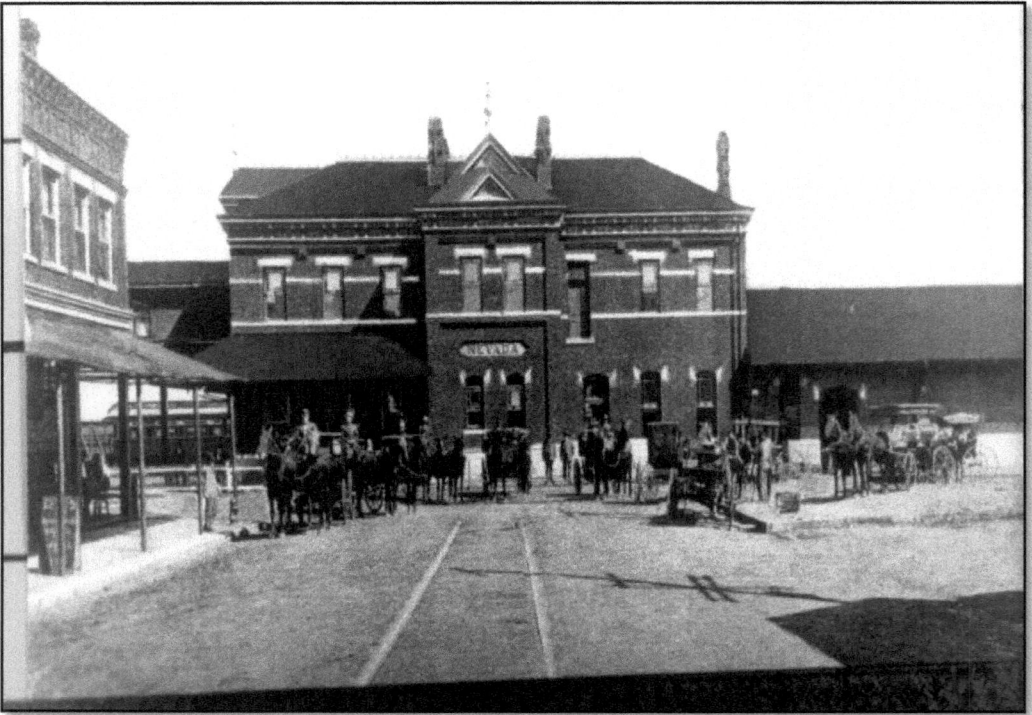

Union Station, Nevada, Mo. (approx. 1900)
(Courtesy of the Bushwhacker Museum, Nevada, Mo.)

4
WELTMER INSTITUTE

WHEN LIZZIE'S FATHER arrived at the Nevada Union Depot, he plus others were met by Weltmer representatives. In addition to course advertisements, testimonials, and publications, *Weltmerism* magazine provided instruction for arrival and lodging. Excerpt from 1901 *Weltmerism* magazine:

When you reach Nevada and step off the train, look for a man wearing a silver badge containing the words "Weltmer Infirmary." If you do not see him when getting off the train, step into the waiting room of the depot and watch for him; he passes through the depot after each train leaves. Mr. Duncan will furnish you free transportation to the Weltmer School of Healing and thence to your boarding place.

Board and lodging ranging from $3.50 to $10.00 per week was also listed in the magazine, plus assistance with boarding locations and free carriage rides to and from the institute for those

WELTMERISM 1901
State Historical Society of Missouri
(SHSMO) artifact
(Courtesy of the Bushwhacker Museum, Nevada, Mo.)

unable to walk. Treatment costs varied from $1.00[h] per office visit to a weekly rate of $5.00 for six treatments. If the patient preferred treatment in their room, the cost was doubled: $2.00 for one session or $10.00 for a week. Home Treatments (Absent Treatments) were $5.00 for one month. No home treatment would be taken for less than one month. Lizzie's father secured affordable lodging offsite and signed up for the $1.00 office visit. But what could his thoughts have been when he first entered the institute?

Excerpts from "Open House" at Weltmer Institute, *Nevada Daily Mail, January 13, 1900:* (Courtesy of the Bushwhacker Museum archives.)

The lecture room is beautiful, being all in blue, other walls are tinted in pale blue shading to a deeper tint to the ceiling and bordered with frescoing[i] in conventional design in blue and white. The room is lighted with hundreds of tiny electric lights, making an indescribably lovely scene.

The American School of Magnetic Healing, known throughout the world, is located in Nevada, the progressive city of Southwest Missouri. The city enjoys the very best climate, both pleasant and healthful, it being located just where the northern and southern climates meet. Navigation is on the main lines of the great Missouri, Kansas, and Texas railroad and the L. and S. division of the Missouri Pacific.

The beautiful and stately building at the corner of Austin and Ash Streets was purchased by Prof. Weltmer and Prof. Kelly, and here they made the home of the American Institute of Magnetic Healing. Several months ago, Prof. Welmer and Prof. Kelly realized that the institution was growing so rapidly and the magnitude of their business was so great that their institute would soon be incapacitated. They at once began to employ architects to draw plans for a large addition.

At a great cost this new addition was added, which makes this building one of the largest and most elegant institutions of this state. This

---

[h] $1 about $36 in today's money.
[i] Fresco—a technique of painting water-based paint on wet plaster.

new building is a three-story structure built upon the most modern plan and fitted throughout with all the modern improvements. The second floor of the structure is divided into many rooms to be used as operating apartments in the treating of patients, all of which are fitted with cold and hot water, steam pipes, and elegantly furnished. The basement of this large addition is arranged for giving Turkish baths and there is no more convenient bathrooms in the state than these.

The third floor occupying the entire length of the building is the spacious and elegant lecture room. Handsome opera chairs have been placed in this department for the convenience of the students. [1]

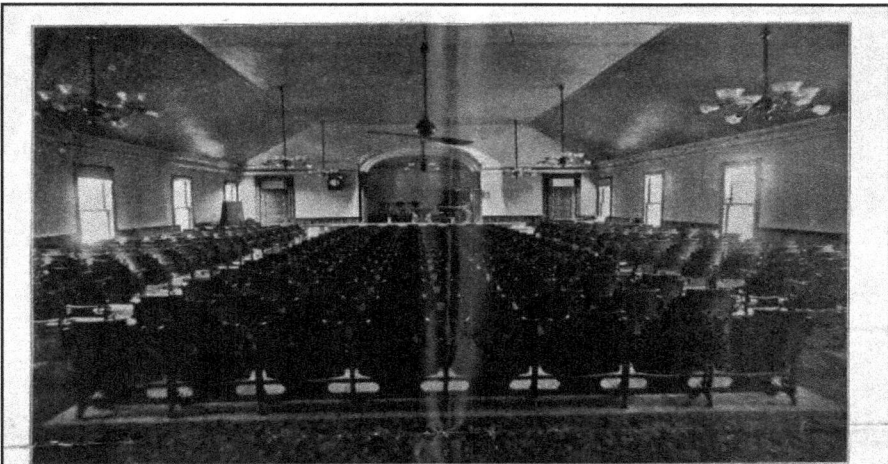

Weltmer Institute Lecture Hall (400 seating capacity)
State Historical Society of Missouri (SHSMO) artifact
Weltmer Journal (Special Edition Vol X, No. XIV, 1906)
(Courtesy of the Bushwhacker Museum, Nevada, Mo.)

During off times, the students and patients were allowed use of the lecture hall for social gatherings, which included the piano located on stage.

The seventeen-room mansion that Sidney Weltmer had procured in 1898 also functioned as a boarding house for patients who purchased a ten-day, stay-for-a-course treatment, charging $100 [j] for this service. Lizzie's father would not have signed up for this treatment plan, but he was treated at the facility for his chronic colitis, which would have fallen under dysentery. It is unknown how many treatments he had, but he was so impressed with the therapeutics that he enrolled in the class courses to become a Professor of Magnetic Healing. Treatments were included.

THE *WELTERMISM* publication advertised the class courses at a reduced cost of $50.00, previously $100.00. The rationale was that the enlarged lecture hall could now accommodate more students and lower the cost for all. Oral Instruction and Practical Demonstration was included with two lectures a day delivered by Professor Weltmer and his specially selected staff. Each student received a text book, a complete mail course, a copy of the *Mystery Revealed* book, office treatments, and a diploma. The class-course students were not limited to four weeks and could remain until they were satisfied with their grasp of the subject. [2]

For $65, students were guaranteed that they would thoroughly master the course in four weeks. It is unknown if extra hands-on sessions were offered to meet this guarantee, but as a result of some extra training, Lizzie's father became proficient in hypnotizing. When he opened his practice, he listed it as a specialty.

In addition to the pride, profit, and prestige of being a Weltmer graduate, Weltmer stated that the graduate had an invaluable advantage of close touch with the institute and benefited from the thousands of dollars the institute spent in advertising Weltmerism.

THE AUDITORIUM courses ran Monday through Saturday starting at 8:00 a.m. to 6:00 p.m. The students entered in and out throughout the day between classes. Specialized sessions covering the same subjects were also offered singly or in smaller groups by appointment only from 7:30 a.m. to 10:00 p.m. each day. The Resident classes followed a similar format to the Extension Course outline:

---

[j] About $3,600 in today's money.

- *Monday*—Scientific Magnetic Massage of the Back.
- *Tuesday*—Scientific Magnetic Massage of the Lower Limb, which included the back and front of the lower limb and the foot. Plus, injuries from infantile paralysis and sciatic neuritis.[k]
- *Wednesday*—Scientific Magnetic Massage of the Upper Limb: massage of muscles and joints and the hands, with the purpose of relieving joints in arthritis and treatment of neuritis.
- *Thursday*—Scientific Magnetic Massage of the Chest and Abdomen. This encompassed the anatomy of the chest, abdomen, and massage for constipation, and healing of the abdominal organs.
- *Friday*—Scientific Magnetic Massage and Anatomy of the neck and head. Massage and healing for throat ailments, eyes and ears were included in the session.

Thursday's session, Scientific Magnetic Massage of the Chest and Abdomen (pictured), was one of the treatments that Lizzie's father would have received for his chronic colitis.

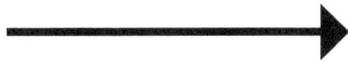

Prof. Weltmer and Associate Performing Abdominal Treatments
(Courtesy of Bushwhacker Museum, Nevada, Mo.)

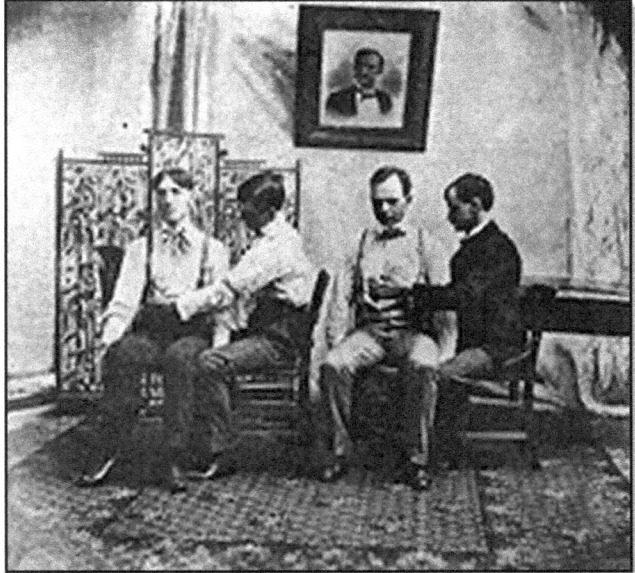

---

[k] Neuritis—inflammation of a nerve.

- *Saturday*—Scientific Suggestion Therapy, Magnetic Healing, and Psycho-therapy—the basic fundamentals of healing combined with other methods to achieve the best results. The consecration of the healer's hands often embraced blessings that were performed before starting all procedures.

STARTING AT 9:00 A.M. each day, half-hour healing services were offered in a darkened room where actual patients or students would lie on the treatment tables or sit in the chairs while others observed. The teacher rarely chose the subject beforehand, his mind had to be sensitized to the thoughts and needs of those before him. Some mornings, the healer would perform an absent treatment, guided to the need of someone far in distance, but present in spirit.

At the beginning of each session, students were reminded that the teachings were universal. Everyone who attended, physically and spiritually, was blessed according to their ability to receive. It was also stressed that the Weltmer healer was a "true healer", not a doctor nor a diagnostician, but by the power of the awakened consciousness of the Kingdom within. [3]

AFTER GRADUATION, some Weltmer students opened practices near the institute. With so many people arriving daily, these new healers would likely snag incoming patients by advertising treatments at reduced rates. With any major decision, monetary or not, it is known that Lizzie's father always studied the situation before moving forward. Before signing up for a resident professor course that cost a good sum of money, it is believed that he visited several of these offsite healers to discuss their format, office setup, and evaluate their skills. He may have even opted for treatments.

CALL UI **Stephenson, The Druggist,** East S of Squa

168   WALLIN, SHAFFER & CO.'S NEVADA CITY DIRECTORY.

Magnetic Healers

American School, 206 S Ash
Consolidated School, 624 E Cherry
Eureka School, 128½ N Cedar
Graves Lena F Mrs, 317 E Cherry
Harpold Grant, 308 W Cherry
Hutchens Sarah G Mrs, 630 E Austin
McCary Mary Miss, 426 W Walnut
Marmaduke Institute, 128 S Main
Missouri Schoof, 121½ W Cherry
National School, 212½ W Cherry
Nevada School, 308 W Cherry
Stanhope Sanitarium. 507 E Cherry
Thurman Joseph C, 609½ E Cherry
Universal Institute, 113½ N Main
Vito-Magnetic Sanitarium, 530 E Cherry

1900-1901 NEVADA CITY DIRECTORY
(Courtesy of the Bushwhacker Museum, Nevada, Mo.)

After completion of the Weltmer Resident Course, Professor W.B. Wilson received his official diploma as a graduate of the S.A. Weltmer School of Healing, August 14, 1900.

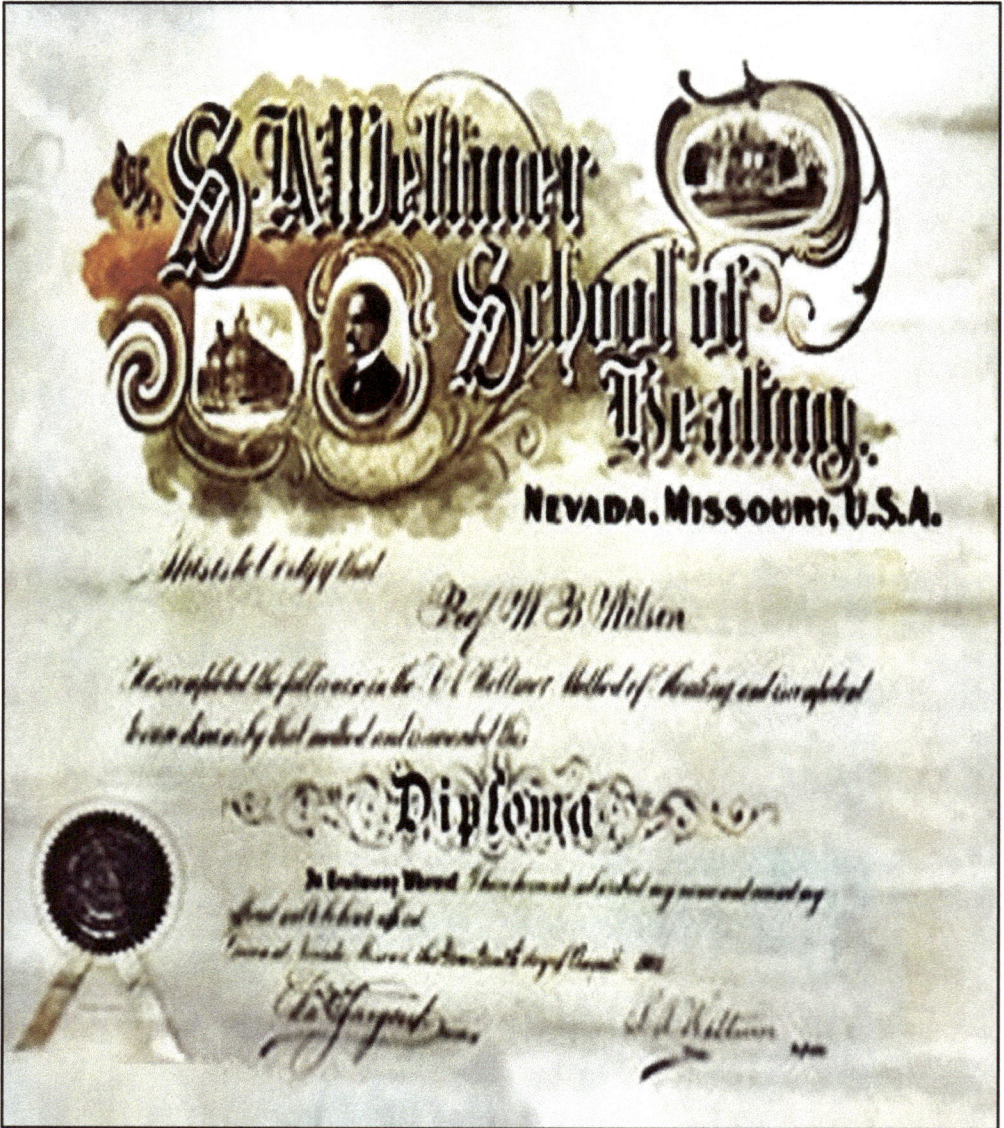

PROFESSOR W.B. WILSON DIPLOMA
August 14, 1900
Signed by S.A. Weltmer
(Author's collection)

5
93 MARKET STREET
Aberdeen, WA

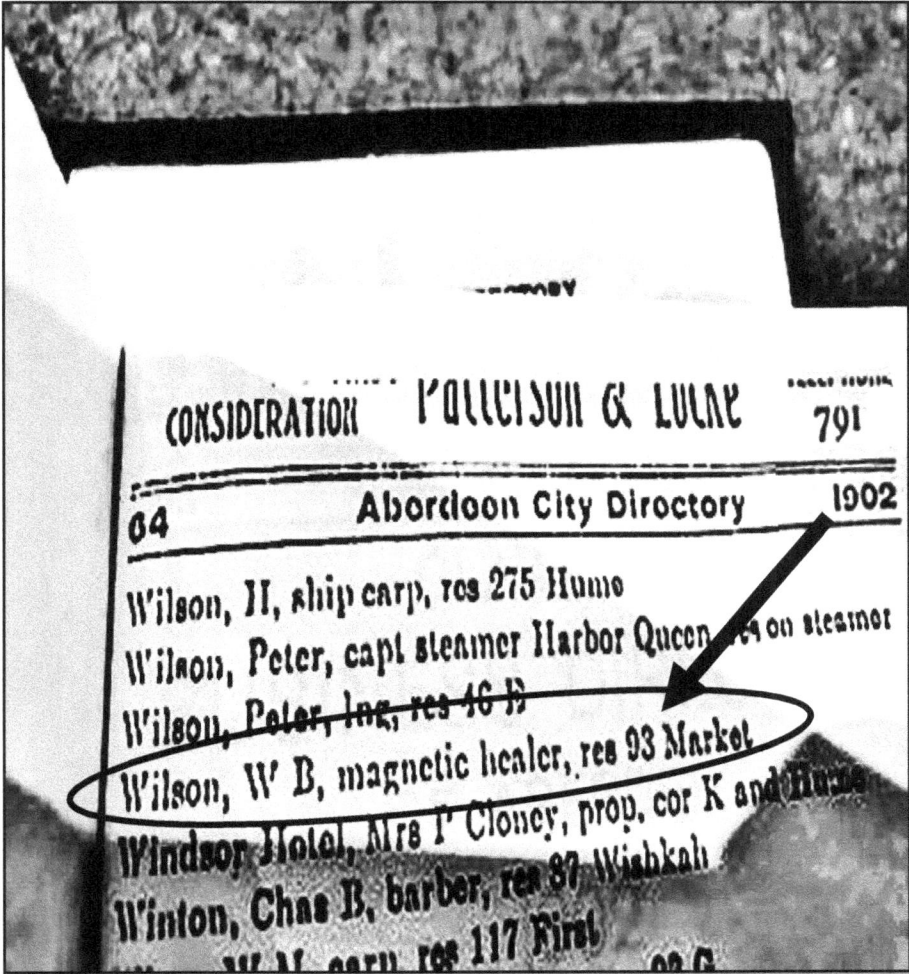

1902 ABERDEEN DIRECTORY
(Courtesy of Polson Museum, Hoquiam, WA)

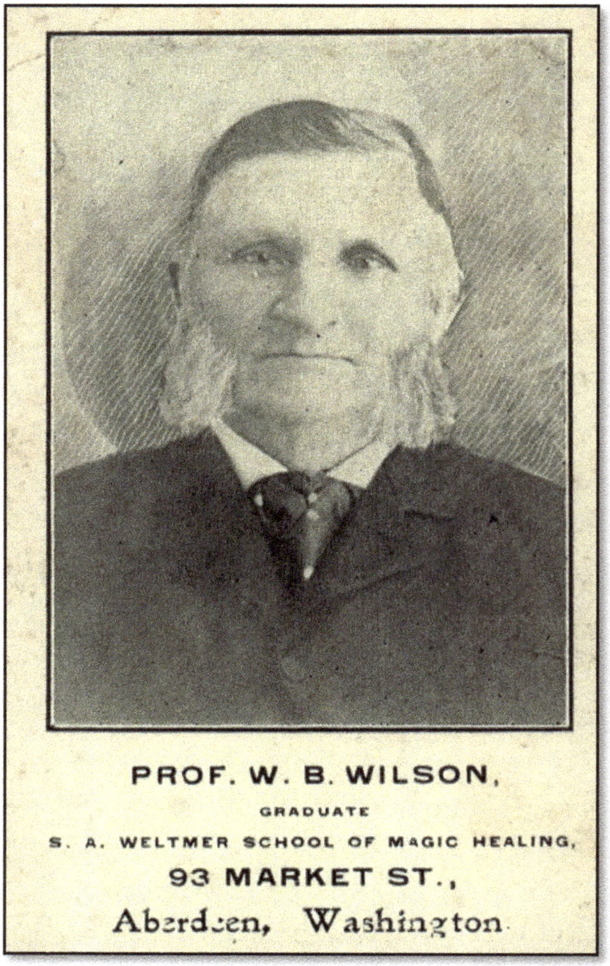

PROF. W. B. WILSON,
GRADUATE
S. A. WELTMER SCHOOL OF MAGIC HEALING,
93 MARKET ST.,
Aberdeen, Washington.

PROFESSOR W.B. WILSON
Magic Healer
(Author's collection)

IN EARLY 1901, LIZZIE'S FATHER had purchased a small house at 93 Market Street, Aberdeen, WA, for his healing practice. With his carpentry skills, he remodeled the building. The Weltmer Institute later published a book in 1912 titled, *How to Succeed*, which included step-by-step instructions. In the early years, students would have received the catalog of the same name covering this criterion.[1]

Essentials listed included a well-cushioned table with illustrations on how to build one. Other required items: stools, muslin sheets and feather pillows. Advice was also given, such as pillow slips must be scrupulously clean and changed often, and toilet facilities with a nearby mirror and folding screen had to be available for patients. Wall paper was to be a small design and mild colored like light blue or light green. Window shades pure white inside and green outside and the curtains always white. In buying chairs, it was best to have one large, elegant, comfortable chair rather than two not-as-nice, and no tuft upholstery furniture. A reception hall or room was a must and had to have a flat-top desk and locking drawers, plus plain office chairs and settees. Two rocking chairs, two straight chairs, and one or two padded foot rests were also suggested, and all articles of wood furniture were recommended to be the same. With Professor Wilson's limited budget, items were donated by family or friends or procured from the secondhand store. Most of the interior design was handled by Lizzie.

WHILE LIZZIE WAS helping in her father's healing practice, she'd travel to Aberdeen by streetcar. She was especially needed when he was treating female patients. One of Weltmer's prerequisites listed in the *How to Succeed* book stated: "When treating a woman, the male practitioner should require the attendance of a relative or a nurse."[1]

Lizzie was organized and a good financier as stated in John Snyder's 1894 letter and the perfect one to oversee her father's bookkeeping and assist at the reception desk. During downtimes, she would study his medical books.

Whenever Professor W.B. Wilson performed treatments, Lizzie assisted with prayer, and if the patient allowed, she would follow her father's instruction and administer procedures, such as: laying on of hands. When he had traveled to Tacoma for court, he put Lizzie in charge of his practice.

---

[1] *How to Succeed*, old catalog (est. date 1897) by Tracy Carleton Weltmer, S.A. Weltmer's son.

On June 9, 1904, Professor Wilson sent his wife, Mary, a letter and wrote the following on the back of the envelope: "Tell Lizzie to treat patents [sic] (patients), but no hypnosis."

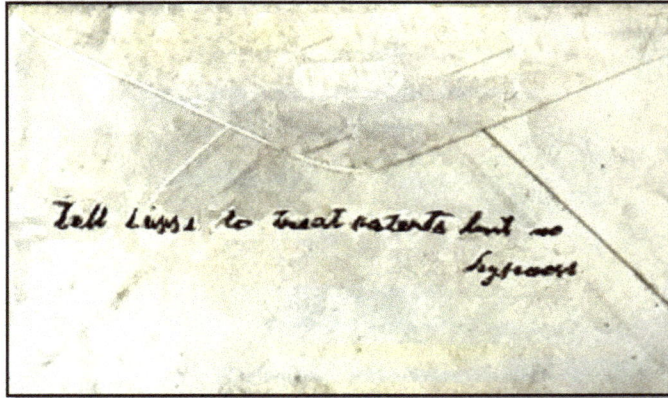

Lizzie's father was an expert hypnotist. He tried to teach Lizzie, but she never mastered the skill. The hypnotic operator (healer) had to possess a dominant, imperial will and self-reliance, self-confidence, and a determination to succeed.

The power of mental concentration was key as it required the power to fix and hold one's attention for extended periods of time. Weltmer regarded this as a natural gift, but also felt with persistent training in concentration, it could be achieved.[2] Lizzie's father was a natural.

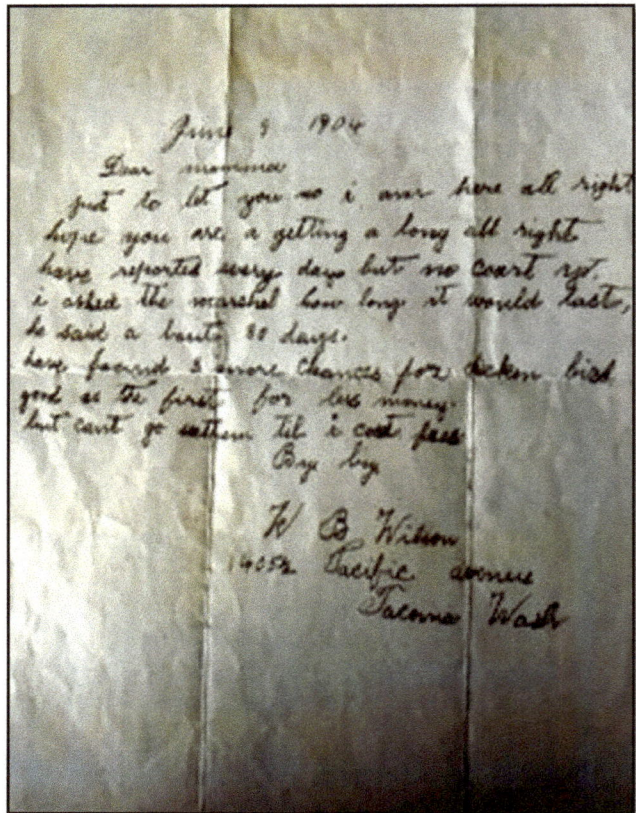

W.B. Wilson 1904 Letter
Tacoma, WA for court
(Author's collection)

44

One experiment that Weltmer listed in the study guide was the grouping of six or seven people for hypnosis. This original study guide, dated 1900, was saved in Lizzie's belongings. The healer would step behind one of the subjects, run his fingers lightly over the person's shoulder and suggest that this person had fleas on him or that water was pouring down his back, or any other idea that the healer wished to suggest. Another experiment was to describe an imaginary line on the floor in front of the subject and tell him he could not step over it. He might be able to fall over it, but could not get his feet over it.

Excerpt from the caption: "The photo shows two positions of the subject and operator (healer). In the first position, the subject's eyes are fixed upon the point of a pencil. In the second position, the subject is reclining with eyes centered on the operator's finger. In both positions, the suggestion given was sleep."[3]

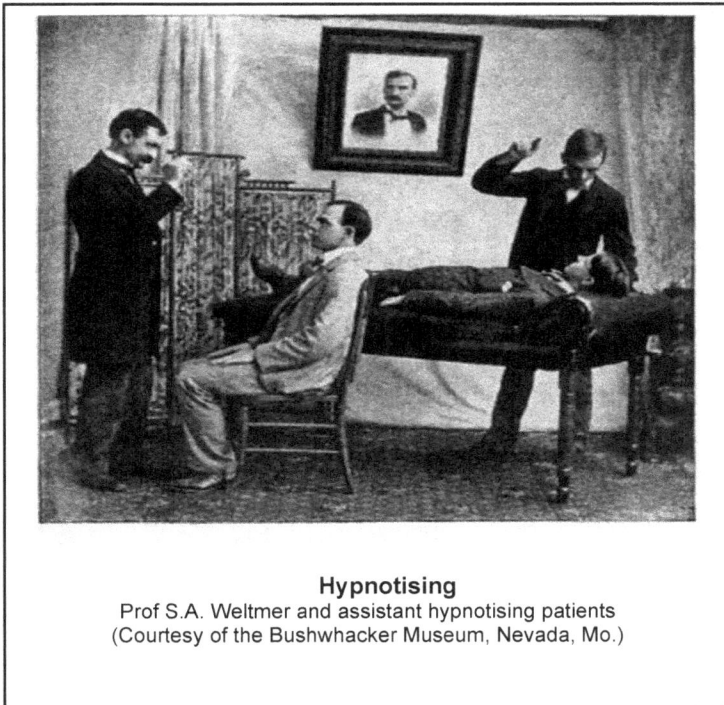

Hypnotising
Prof S.A. Weltmer and assistant hypnotising patients
(Courtesy of the Bushwhacker Museum, Nevada, Mo.)

Professor Wilson practiced on family and friends and perfected several hypnotic experiments, plus prayed and meditated to enhance his concentration. The fact that his stature commanded respect as did his confidence and strong belief in God, most of those he performed his hypnosis on followed his commands. He was so confident in his skill that he handed out Professional Hypnotist cards specific to this service.

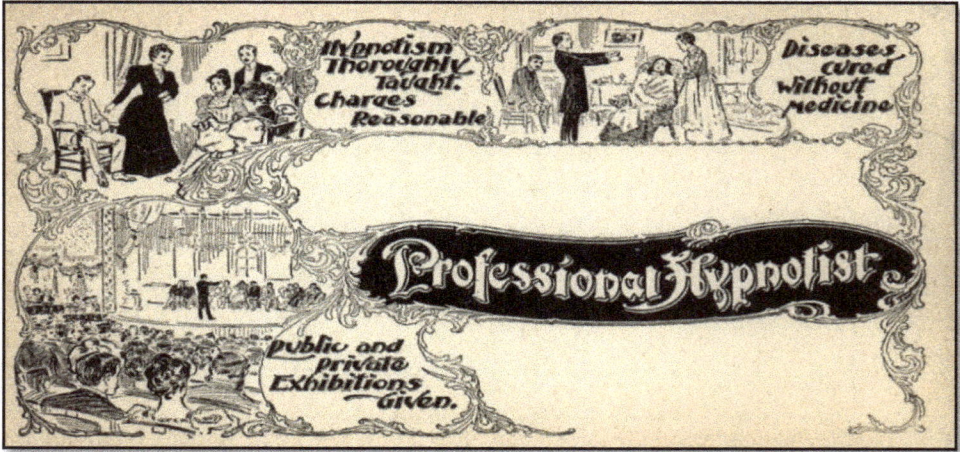

**PROF. W. B. WILSON'S,
PROFESSIONAL HYPNOTIST CARD**
(Author's collection)

The patient's name, date, and appointment time would be written in the blank spaces. It is unknown what he charged, but Lizzie tracked the schedule. All public sessions were in the evenings and she was always at his side and would spend the night at his office after an event.

To achieve a hypnotic state, the healer had to place the patient under his control, first with trust and then specific instruction and positive suggestion. The Weltmer doctrine for hypnosis was that both minds had to be in agreement. One positive and the other passive or receptive. The stronger the positiveness of the operator (healer) and receptiveness of the patient, the quicker and deeper the hypnotic influence.[4] It was also believed that strong-willed personalities, not weak-minded or nervous people, were the most receptive, based on the theory that no one could be hypnotized against one's own will.

THE WELTMER METHOD OF MAGNETIC HEALING.

ORIGINATED BY _____

PROF. S. A. WELTMER.

(COPYRIGHTED 1897.)

_____

LETTER NO. 2.

HYPNOTISM.

METHODS OF MESMERIZING.

Before you can place a person under your control, you must have secured his undivided attention. Suppose you want to fix a person's eyes. Assume a position about five feet in front of the person who is to be the subject; close all of your fingers on your right hand except the first two; have the subject fix his eyes on the ends of those two fingers, and move slowly toward him telling him that when you reach a point about four inches from his eyes, to close them; then tell him positively that his eyes are closed and that he cannot open them. If the subject is at all passive, he will take this suggestion, and if he takes it, he will take any other suggestion.

TO HYPNOTIZE WITHOUT CLOSING THE EYES: Assume the same position before your subject as above, and advance in the same manner, offering the suggestion that when you reach a point about four inches from his eyes he will take any suggestion you may give. Now, if when you reach that point, the eyes of the subject assume a vacant stare, you may know that he is hypnotized. Now, suggest to him that there is a dog in front of him, and he will see the dog. Or suggest that he is eating fruit of some

Prof. W. B. Wilson's, Pg 1 of 4
"Hypnotism"
Study Guide (1900)
(Author's collection)

LAYING ON OF HANDS was the physical sensation behind which the suggestion entered the unconscious mind undoubted and unchallenged.[5] When combined, it secured the Perfect Agreement, which was considered the arch of Weltmerism.[6] Weltmer often cited Matthew 18:19: "Again, I tell you, if two of you on earth agree (harmonize together, make a symphony together) about whatever (anything and everything) they may ask, it will come to pass and be done for them by My Father in heaven."[7]

The purpose of the two was to produce "Vital Magnetism", which was the vibrations of the healer's nervous system felt in the patient. Laying on of Hands was the intricate part of healing and had to be perfected to achieve positive results. It was the most practiced treatment at the institute. Hypnosis was a strong asset for a healer, but many students lacked the confidence or ability to perfect it, as in Lizzie's case, so Laying on of Hands with the Power of Suggestion became the crux of their healing.

Lizzie's father relied on it as well. Many patients didn't want to be hypnotized, and those who did in group or public settings, did so for its entertainment purposes too. Professor Wilson enjoyed his hypnosis seminars, whether for teaching or entertainment, didn't matter as long as it resulted in healing a patient or breaking a bad habit.

With Laying on of Hands, students were taught that animal magnetism, also known as mesmerism, was the invisible natural force possessed by all living things. Electro-biology/Electrical Psychology extended to the philosophy of disease. Weltmer believed that the connecting link between mind, matter, and blood circulation was voluntary and involuntary powers of the mind, and was the foundation of the nervous system. His theory was that blood circulation had two systems: arterial blood, which was positive and venous blood, negative. As the blood moved by forces of electricity, taken in at the lung's inspiration, that diseases in the body didn't originate in the blood but were in the electricity of the nerves. With these philosophies, he stressed to his students that the Laying on of Hands was one of the key elements of healing. Lizzie's father never deviated from these teachings. Nor did Lizzie.

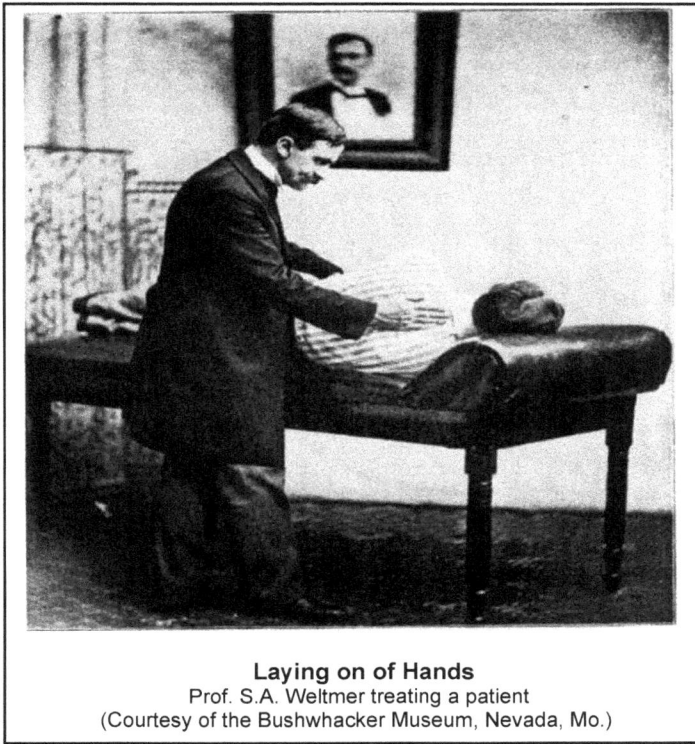

Laying on of Hands
Prof. S.A. Weltmer treating a patient
(Courtesy of the Bushwhacker Museum, Nevada, Mo.)

In order for the sensation to be most effective, it was deemed necessary to heat the hands. Weltmer outlined a process: Raise arms to right angles, projecting sideways, then from the wrist let the hands hang limp. After several seconds, tense all the muscles of the arm, drop the hands by the sides, and feel the blood rush down. The final step was to breathe upon the palms to impart a slight moisture and rub the hands briskly. Now with the hands warmed, the physical sensation would be more noticeable to the patient and enable the suggestion to reach the unconscious mind without being doubted, denied, or challenged. [8]

Weltmer outlined specific treatment regions:

- The Cervical Plexus controlled the organs of the head, eyes, nose, ears, and tongue.
- The Brachial Plexus controlled the arms and the shoulders.
- Nerves from the Dorsal Plexus controlled the throat, lungs, heart, spleen, liver, and intestines.
- The Lumbar Plexus treated lumbago. The Sacral Plexus the limbs and pelvic organs.

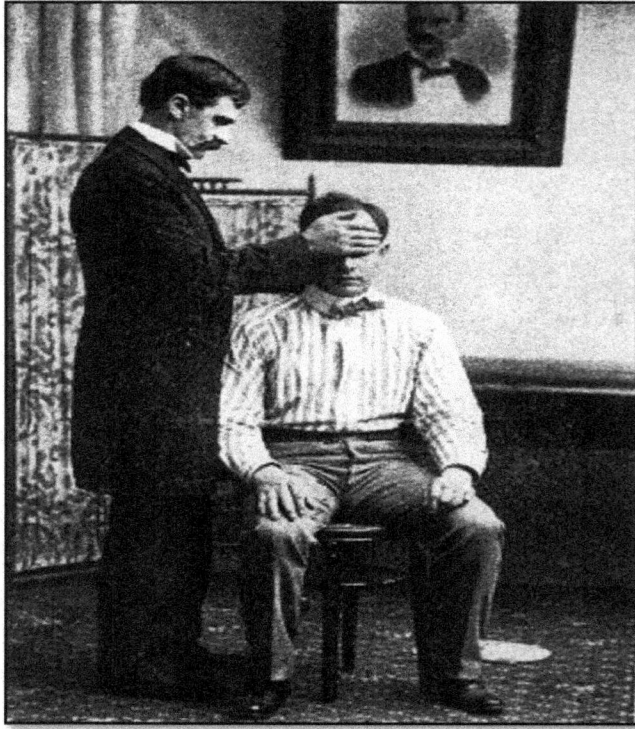

Laying on of Hands
Prof. S.A. Weltmer treating a patient with nasal problems
(Cervical Plexus region)
(Courtesy of the Bushwhacker Museum, Nevada, Mo.)

Another treatment method was called imparted motion. By laying the right hand on the plexus of the organ to be treated, the healer would then contract the biceps with a gentle, quivering motion. He'd ask the patient if he felt it. The patient would reply, "yes." While the attention of both the conscious and unconscious mind was focused on this motion, the suggestion by the healer would be that these vibrations were restoring healthy activity, which would lodge in the unconscious mind and do its work.

THE WELTMER METHOD OF MAGNETIC HEALING.

ORIGINATED BY ——

PROF. S. A. WELTMER.

(COPYRIGHTED 1897.)

LETTER NO. 4.

VITAL MAGNETISM.

THE LAYING ON OF HANDS.

If you will put your hand on a person's back between the shoulders, exercising the intention of making him feel the vibrations from your hand, about three out of five will feel the effect of it. Or, if you will take both hands of a person in your hands, placing the thumb of your right hand between the third and fourth fingers on the back of the person's left hand, the left hand the same--your left hand on the person's right hand, and exercise an intention to send a current or vibration through your right hand into the left hand of the person, he will feel a perceptible current steal up the left arm as if coming from an electric battery. The feeling you produce is what is called Vital Magnetism. The process of making the vibrations of your nervous system felt in the nervous system of another person is called Vital Magnetism. This has been called by various names. Prof. Antone Mesmer called it Magnetism. Deleuze called it Animal Magnetism. Dodd called it Electro-Biology and Electrical Psychology. Later writers and investigators have concluded that the best term for this mysterious force is to call it Vital Magnetism. A great many persons are so susceptible to this influence that if you will pass your hand down in front of the face,

**Prof. W. B. Wilson's
"Laying on of Hands"
Study Guide (1900)**
(Author's collection)

51

THE POWER OF SUGGESTION in healing followed in line with hypnosis and laying on of hands. "Inspire your patient a belief in his own strength, encourage him to trust himself, to rely on himself, to eat and breathe, and drink for the purpose of bringing into his life health and casting disease out of his body."[9]

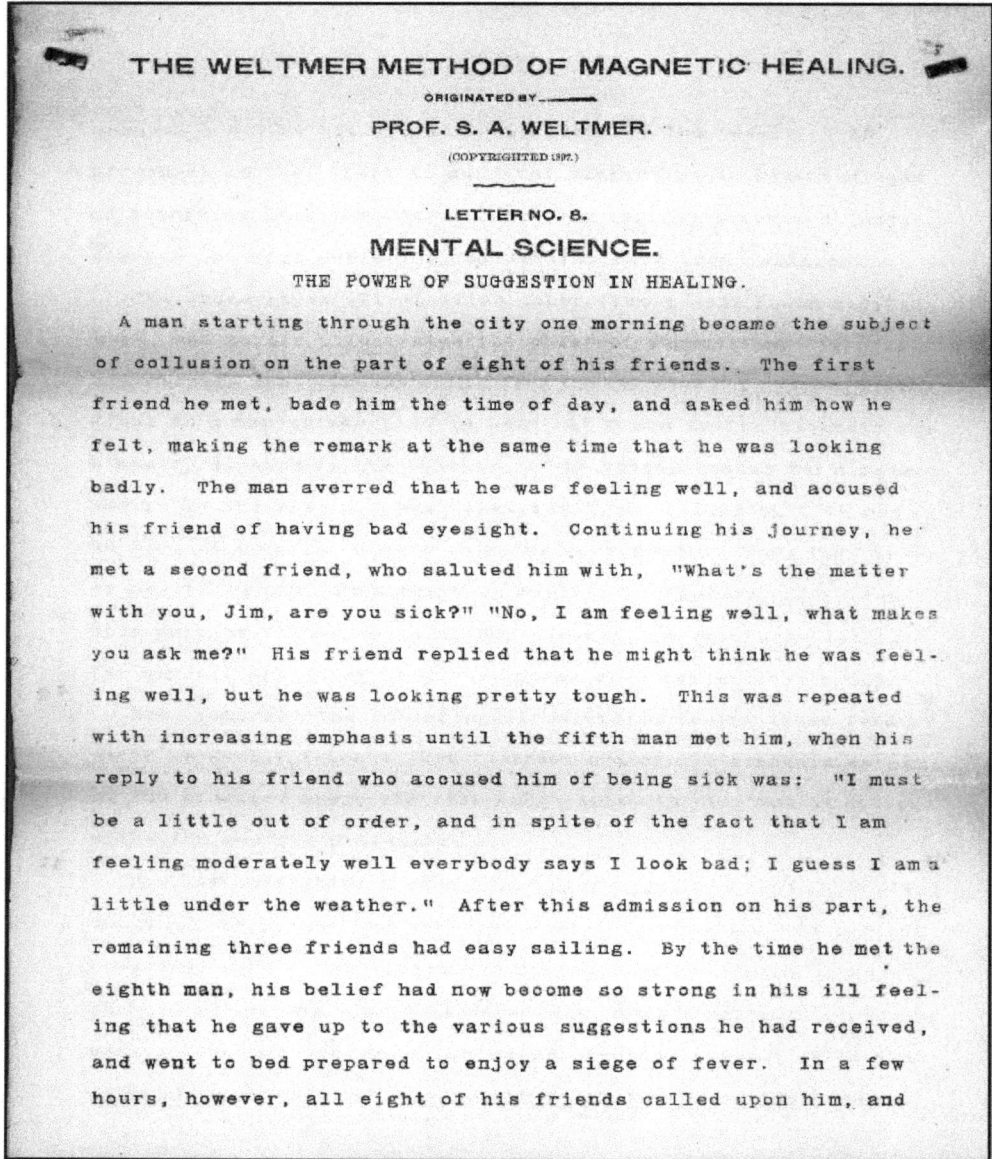

THE WELTMER METHOD OF MAGNETIC HEALING.

ORIGINATED BY

PROF. S. A. WELTMER.

(COPYRIGHTED 1897.)

LETTER NO. 8.

MENTAL SCIENCE.

THE POWER OF SUGGESTION IN HEALING.

A man starting through the city one morning became the subject of collusion on the part of eight of his friends. The first friend he met, bade him the time of day, and asked him how he felt, making the remark at the same time that he was looking badly. The man averred that he was feeling well, and accused his friend of having bad eyesight. Continuing his journey, he met a second friend, who saluted him with, "What's the matter with you, Jim, are you sick?" "No, I am feeling well, what makes you ask me?" His friend replied that he might think he was feeling well, but he was looking pretty tough. This was repeated with increasing emphasis until the fifth man met him, when his reply to his friend who accused him of being sick was: "I must be a little out of order, and in spite of the fact that I am feeling moderately well everybody says I look bad; I guess I am a little under the weather." After this admission on his part, the remaining three friends had easy sailing. By the time he met the eighth man, his belief had now become so strong in his ill feeling that he gave up to the various suggestions he had received, and went to bed prepared to enjoy a siege of fever. In a few hours, however, all eight of his friends called upon him, and

**Prof. W. B. Wilson's
"Power of Suggestion"
Study Guide (1900)**
(Author's collection)

DESIRE. Weltmer emphasized this as prayer, faith, and procreation. That we were taught to pray, to desire, to let our wants to be known, to ask, and to believe. And that the human mind could not desire a thing that did not exist.

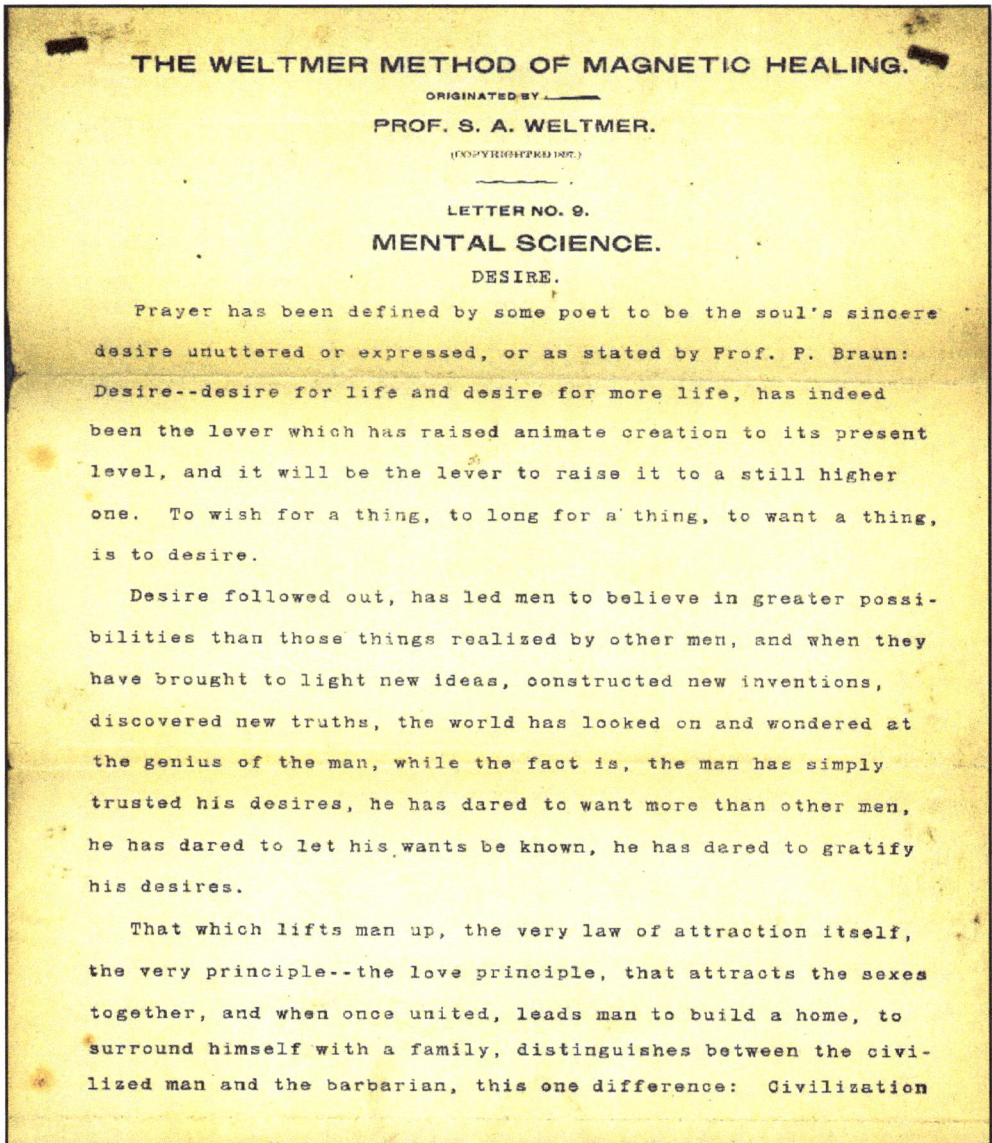

THE WELTMER METHOD OF MAGNETIC HEALING.

ORIGINATED BY

PROF. S. A. WELTMER.

(COPYRIGHTED 1897.)

LETTER NO. 9.

MENTAL SCIENCE.

DESIRE.

Prayer has been defined by some poet to be the soul's sincere desire unuttered or expressed, or as stated by Prof. P. Braun: Desire--desire for life and desire for more life, has indeed been the lever which has raised animate creation to its present level, and it will be the lever to raise it to a still higher one. To wish for a thing, to long for a thing, to want a thing, is to desire.

Desire followed out, has led men to believe in greater possibilities than those things realized by other men, and when they have brought to light new ideas, constructed new inventions, discovered new truths, the world has looked on and wondered at the genius of the man, while the fact is, the man has simply trusted his desires, he has dared to want more than other men, he has dared to let his wants be known, he has dared to gratify his desires.

That which lifts man up, the very law of attraction itself, the very principle--the love principle, that attracts the sexes together, and when once united, leads man to build a home, to surround himself with a family, distinguishes between the civilized man and the barbarian, this one difference: Civilization

Prof. W. B. Wilson's
"Desire"
Study Guide (1900)
(Author's collection)

It is known that both Lizzie and her father followed this premise throughout their practices. The back of Professor Wilson's business cards outlined his beliefs: "He that believeth on Me, the works that I do shall he do also."

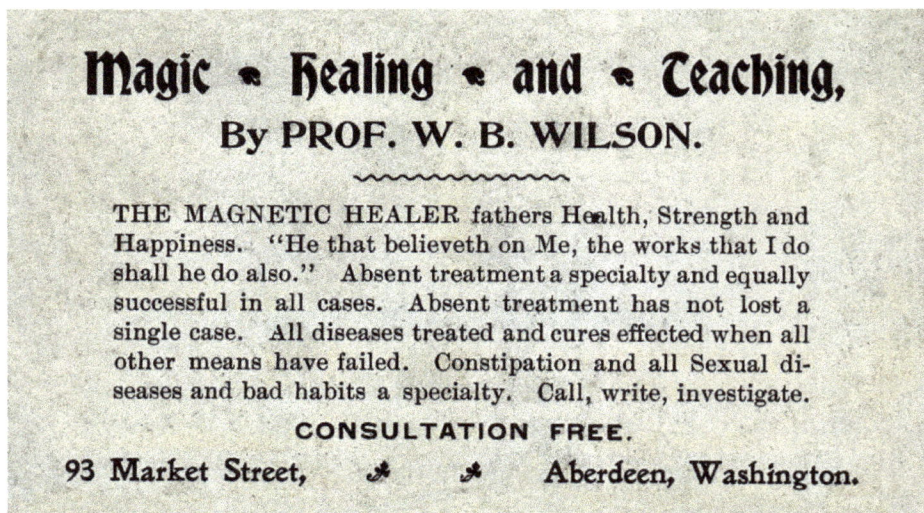

Magic • Healing • and • Teaching,
By PROF. W. B. WILSON.

THE MAGNETIC HEALER fathers Health, Strength and Happiness. "He that believeth on Me, the works that I do shall he do also." Absent treatment a specialty and equally successful in all cases. Absent treatment has not lost a single case. All diseases treated and cures effected when all other means have failed. Constipation and all Sexual diseases and bad habits a specialty. Call, write, investigate.
CONSULTATION FREE.
93 Market Street, ♣ ♣ Aberdeen, Washington.

PROF. W.B. WILSON'S BUSINESS CARD
(Back)
(Author's collection)

LIZZIE'S FATHER started every treatment with prayer. He'd memorize passages from his Bible, and with his deep methodical tone, recite verses often while holding the patient's hands. For special cases, it is known that he'd prepare for hours, same as a minister with his sermon. Many times, Lizzie stepped in to do the prayer. When a patient couldn't come to his office, he'd perform Absent Treatments, which he learned at the Weltmer Institute.

With Absent Treatments, Weltmer believed that space and time had no existence for the spiritual being; they were only necessary conditions of our conscious self. And when vibrations were sent out to a person, who could be thousands of miles away, it was the positive mind transmitting and the passive mind receiving.[10]

Absent Treatment as described in the 1900 *Weltmerism* magazine:

Prof. Weltmer prefers that prospective patients come to his infirmary and take personal treatment, but where for any reason this is impossible, they can be successfully healed in their own homes by the Weltmer

Method of Absent or Home Treatment. Distance or lack of means or strength to travel need be no bar to the relief of anyone afflicted with any disease, no matter what its nature. Thousands of grateful people who have been restored to health and happiness by this Home Treatment gladly testify to its value and efficacy. Its cost is only $5.00 [m] for a month's treatment. [11]

The back of Professor Wilson's business card read: "Absent Treatment a specialty and equally successful in all cases." It is believed that Lizzie handled most of the Absent Treatment paperwork, which included sending out questionnaires to the home-treatment patients. Once her father evaluated the patient's reply, he'd provide written assessments plus a date and time to synchronize minds for the healing process to begin. It is unknown how many Absent Treatments he performed, but must have had some success as Lizzie advertised this service in her own practice years later. A 1918 envelope with her handwriting "Absent Treatments" was among her belongings:

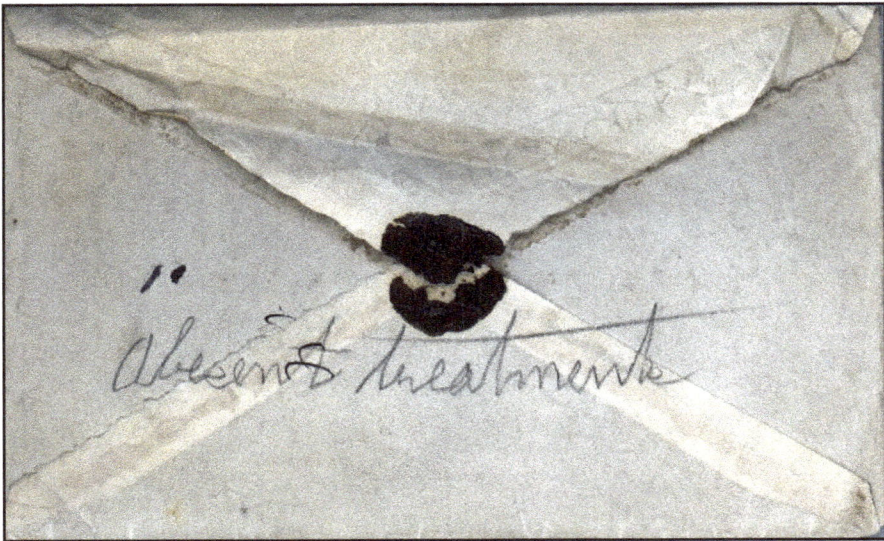

ABSENT TREATMENTS ENVELOPE
In Lizzie's Belongings
Lizzie's handwriting
(Author's collection)

---

[m] About $180 in today's money.

ADVERTISING WAS ONE of the key elements for success. Guidelines were taught in the Weltmer courses and later outlined in his book, *How to Succeed.* Weltmer stressed that personal habits and appearance of good health, plus manner of dress and sincerity in your work were a necessity, but greater than all of these, was the ability to cure the patients. [12]

With Personal habits, he emphasized avoidance of destructive behaviors such as over-eating, drinking alcohol or smoking or chewing tobacco. Even excessive drinking of coffee or tea could overload the body and should be stopped. Personal hygiene too: bathing, care of hands, finger nails, teeth, and hair was a must. Weltmer advised that the practitioner should feel no hesitancy in urging his patients to adopt these good practices too.[13]

Professor W.B. Wilson abided by all of these rules and was never seen in public without a suit. Lizzie also took pride in her professional appearance, but did they encourage their patients to follow these habits? Not likely. Aberdeen and Hoquiam were lumber towns, and those who didn't own businesses or of the professional class, would have more than likely worked as lumberjacks or laborers in the mill, to name several, and would have come straight from work for treatment. Most of the women, however, would have been well-groomed on all their outings.

In addition to word of mouth, Professor Wilson and Lizzie handed out cards during various community events: church bazaars, lodge meetings, and town halls. Even though the Weltmer advertisements stated that Weltmer healers could net as much as $25.00 a day, it is doubtful that Professor Wilson earned that amount. He did, however, make enough to sustain his business, pay himself and Lizzie, and send money to Mary at the homestead. He was so engaged with his practice that he spent most days and nights at the office. Mary's frustration is conveyed in a letter to Lizzie.

Excerpt from 1903 letter: "Papa is downtown where he stays most all the time, only (comes home) when he wants something to eat."[14] (Mary Wilson's letter, 1903, 163.)

6
HOQUIAM

ON OCTOBER 16, 1903, the big fire of Aberdeen destroyed seven city blocks, 140 buildings, and 300 people were left homeless. The estimated damage was over one-half million dollars.[n] Eleven days later, another fire erupted that leveled the commercial district, only blocks away from Professor Wilson's office. The Aberdeen store owners, churches and organizations united to help the displaced and began rebuilding their city. Even though Professor Wilson's building was spared, the fire impacted his practice.

Lizzie's parents relocated to Hoquiam. There were several reasons for this move: reduced business in Aberdeen due to the fire, her mother's loneliness, and Lizzie's desire to become more involved as a healer. Professor Wilson continued to service his Aberdeen patients, but most of his equipment and furnishings had been moved to Lizzie's home. A remodel on Lizzie's house was started and continued over the next few years.

By 1905, Lizzie began taking correspondence courses and had changed her trade name to S.L. Snyder.[o] One of the courses was the Dickson School of Memory.

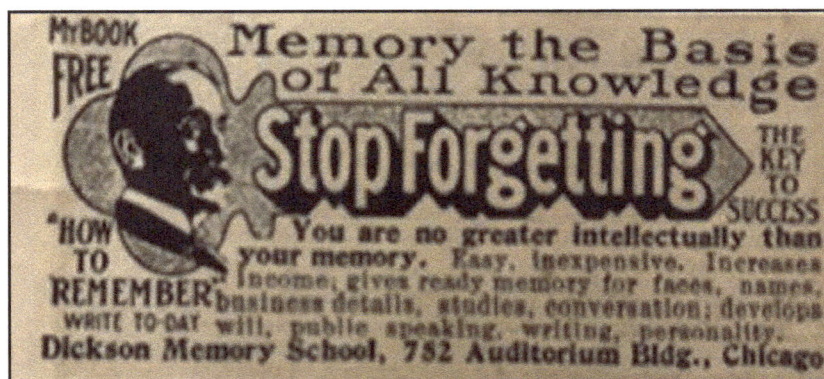

THE DICKSON SCHOOL OF MEMORY AD
(Author's collection)

---

[n] *On the Harbor, From Black Friday to Nirvana*, John C. Hughes & Ryan Teague Beckwith; published 2001, 2005, 2012, 8-13 (Aberdeen's Black Friday).
[o] S.L. Snyder: Sarah LIZZIE (Elizabeth) Snyder (née Wilson).

The advertisements for the memory school: "How to read character," offered a practical course in character analysis. Another advertised: "You are no greater intellectually than your memory. Learn to develop will, concentration, self-confidence, conversation, and public speaking." Prior to opening the memory school in 1900, Henry Dickson (1848-1924) was an instructor in public speaking at the University of Chicago.

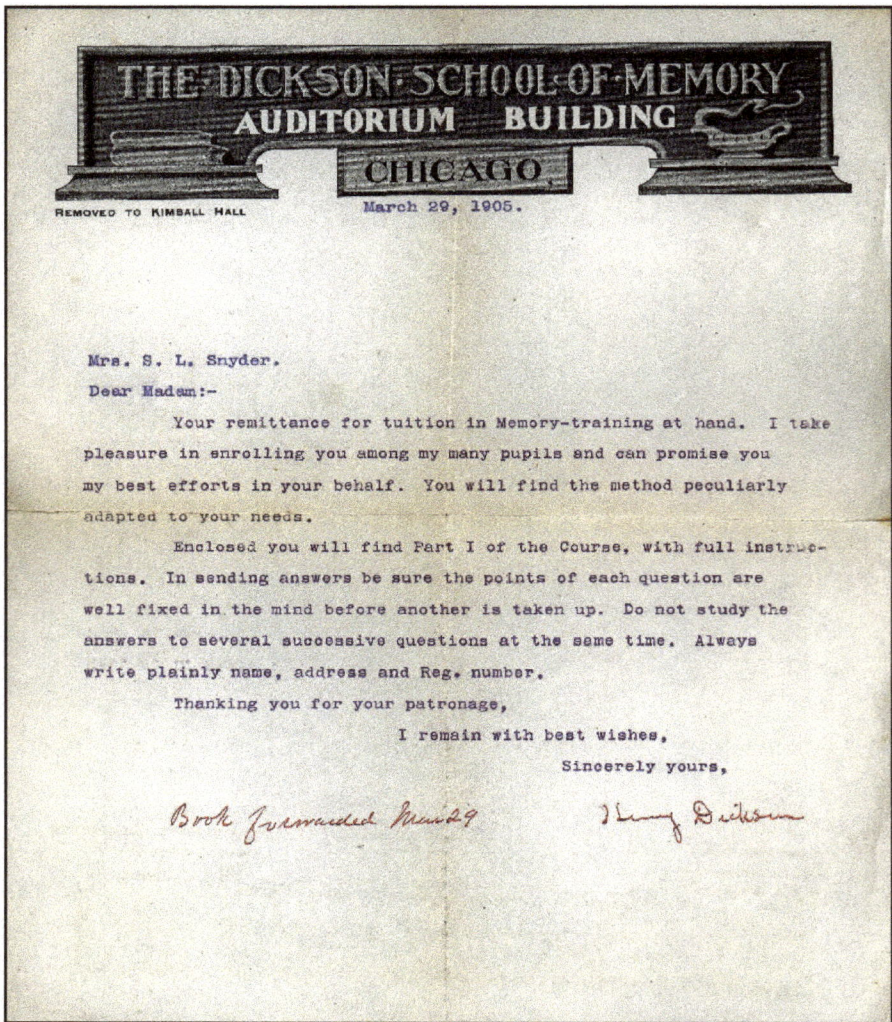

THE DICKSON SCHOOL OF MEMORY
Enrollment Letter (March 29, 1905)
(Author's collection)

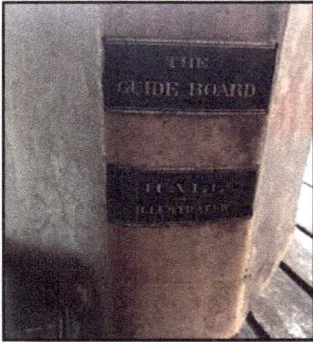

The Guide Board
S.L. Snyder Artifact
(Author's collection)

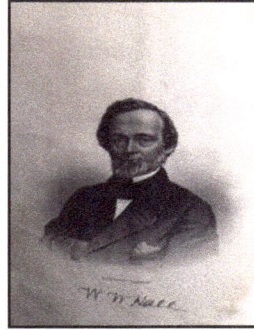

William Whitty Hall
(1810—1876)

LIZZIE BEGAN RESEARCHING other teachings too. One was the 762-page *The Guide Board* book, published in 1872 by Dr. William W. Hall. Dr. Hall believed in healthy living and was described as the forgotten researcher in the field of sleep science.

The Guide Board included illustrations throughout and some of his key messages included: "Men consume too much food, too much medicine, too little pure air and need more outside exercise and proper sleep." He also provided treatments for almost every type of disease known to man.

Regardless of the weather, Dr. Hall believed that hours of daily pure air and outside activity were necessary.

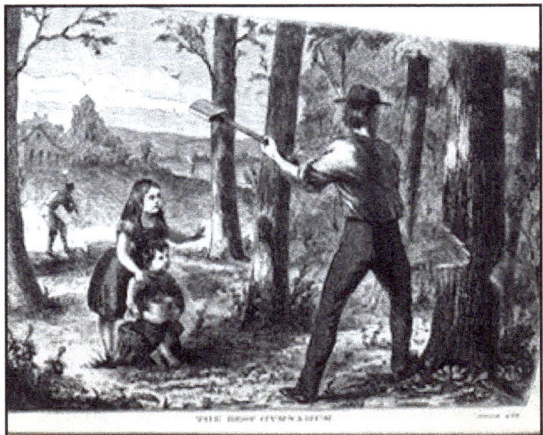

Illustration from book titled:
The Best Gymnasium
(Author's collection)

ANOTHER BOOK found in Lizzie's collection was *Perfect Health,* published in 1901 by Charles C. Haskell. He centered on fitness, healing, medicine, and a new philosophy of "fasting." Haskell, initially a school teacher, went on to become a successful publisher and author. He was known as a health reformer and leading advocate for the fasting cure.

59

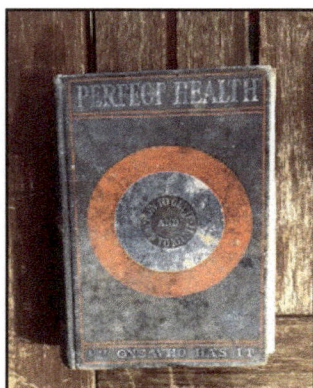

Perfect Health
S.L. Snyder Artifact
(Author's collection)

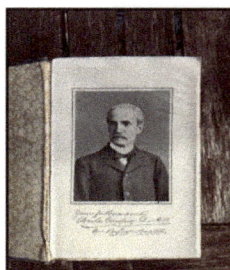

Charles C.
Haskell
(1840—1914)

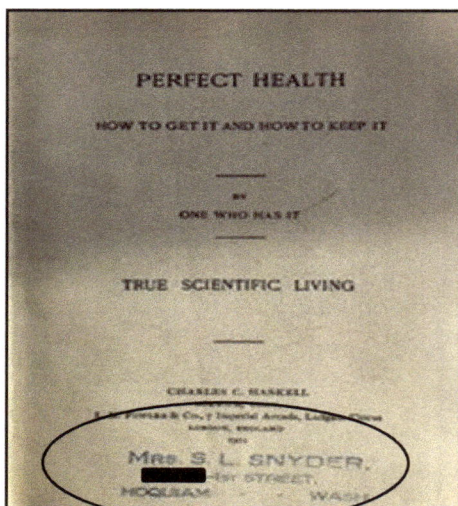

S.L. Snyder Artifact
(Author's collection)

WHILE LIZZIE WAS expanding her knowledge, her father had enrolled in the American College of Mechano-Therapy correspondence course. On August 25, 1909, he earned a diploma and added this new treatment for his patients. Weltmer's Laying on of Hands was a form of this treatment through massage, but mechano-therapy went beyond with actual manipulations of the bones, joints, and muscles. Mechano-Therapy was described as the Practice of Osteopathy, but had elements of chiropractic too.

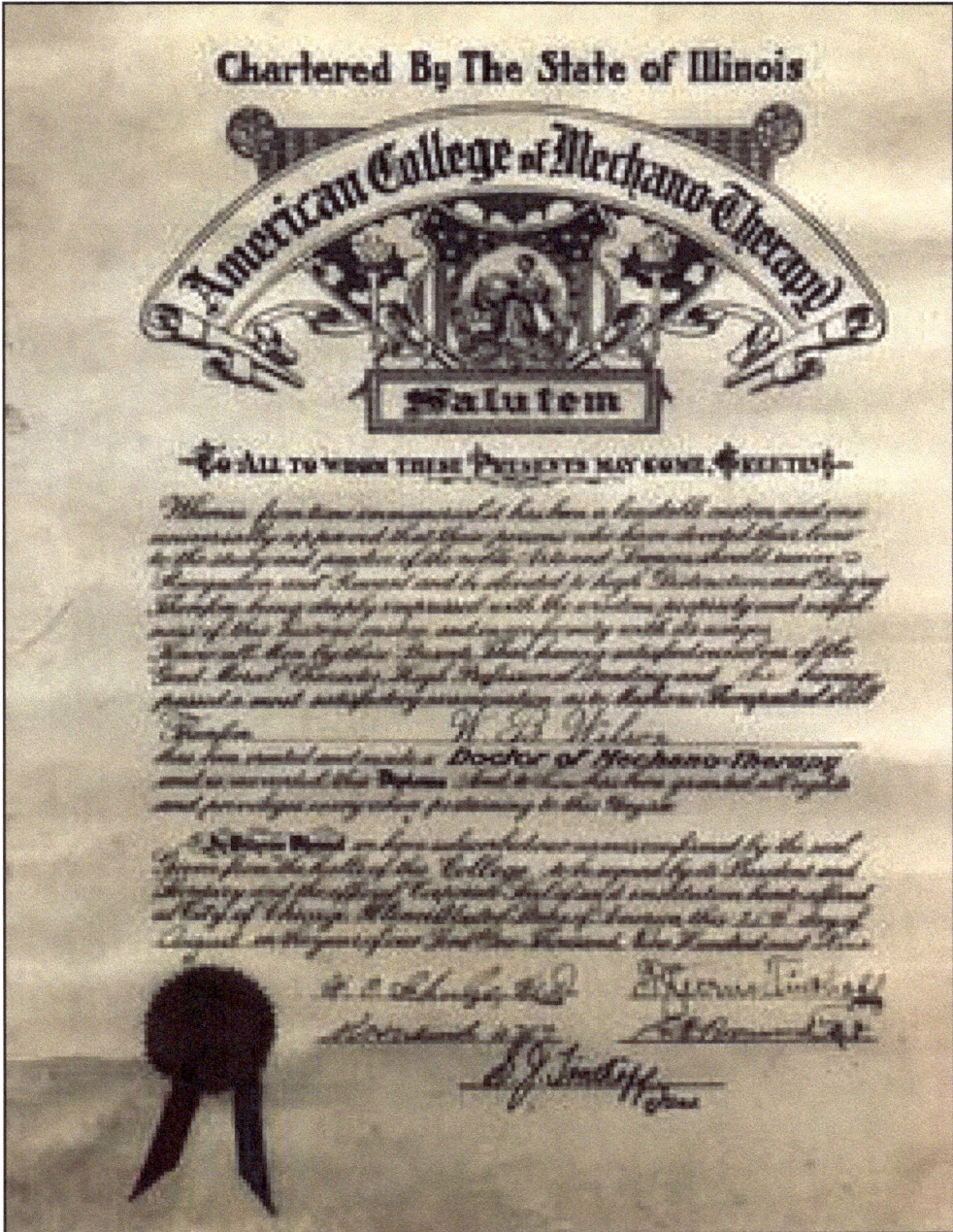

PROFESSOR W.B. WILSON 1909 DIPLOMA
AMERICAN COLLEGE OF MECHANO-THERAPY
(Author's collection)

The Chinese had perfected the art of massage and bone-setting thousands of years before the Christian era, but it was Andrew Taylor Still who was the founder of osteopathic medicine in the United States.[1]

Born in Virginia 1828, Andrew Still was the son of a Methodist minister and a doctor. He farmed, studied medicine in Kansas City, and practiced with his father in the West among the pioneers and Native Americans. As a student, he studied the anatomy of animals, skinning and dissecting. In the early 1850's, he fought with John Brown, an American abolitionist, in the Kansas boarder warfare.

He read medical texts and perfected his knowledge of the human skeletal structure by identifying bones while blindfolded and moved on to the study of muscles, ligaments, and the vascular system. By 1854, he began practicing regular medicine, but there were no medical licensing laws at that time, nor barriers to enter the profession.

Serving in the Civil War as a hospital steward for the Union Army interrupted his studies. He returned to his Kansas medical practice in 1864. Shortly after, three of his children died from an outbreak of Spinal Meningitis despite the noble efforts of several medical colleagues. With his faith in modern medicine eroded, he was driven back to research and determined that prescribing toxic pharmaceuticals was not nature's way of healing.[2] For a period, he practiced as a nomad doctor in Missouri, performing cures with his new science and advertising as a magnetic healer, same as Weltmer had done years later.

Andrew Still built osteopathy on the principle that man was a machine, and when a man became diseased, an expert mechanical engineer (the osteopath) would adjust his machinery. Still had perfected techniques for correction of the skeletal abnormalities. He started with palpitations, first feeling the patient's body for the lesion along with getting a patient's history, blood pressure, and laboratory tests, such as urine analysis. These allowed the osteopath to diagnose the affected organ, deduce what vessels and nerves might be affected, and manipulate corrections with a sensitive touch. When setting a dislocated shoulder, he'd first place a hand at the initial location, and with little force, push the elbow toward the contracted muscles, then rotate the humerus into its socket.

He never used specialized appliances and usually pressed the patient against a chair or a door jamb or any other immovable object that was handy. He often stated, "the osteopathic physician removes the obstruction, and lets Nature's remedy—arterial blood—be the doctor." The creed of the osteopath was simple: "Find it, fix it, and leave it alone." He also believed that God or Nature was the only doctor man should respect, and went on to say, "Osteopathy was God's law." [3]

By 1887, Still resettled in Kirksville, Missouri and began teaching his sons osteopathy. In 1889, he opened an osteopathic infirmary drawing patients to Kirksville by trainload. Three years later, in 1892, he opened the American School of Osteopathy, which provided a four-year course, whose clinics and hospitals drew patients nationwide as well as from Canada. [4] Still, like Weltmer, had no difficulty suggesting surgery when no other options were available. By 1897, he introduced surgery into the Kirksville curriculum, taught by two faculty with orthodox surgical training. [5]

AS OSTEOPATHIC TREATMENTS were gaining popularity, medical doctor, Charles Schulze, stepped into the arena. Schulze, an 1897 graduate of Rush Medical College, had practiced medicine in Illinois, Minnesota, and Wisconsin. He formed the American College of Mechano-Therapy, which operated in Chicago from 1905 through 1920 with Schulze as the president.

Professed as the "largest eclectic school of drugless healing in the world," the American College of Mechano-Therapy published the *Text-book of Osteopathy* (1910), and *Clinical Lectures on Mechano-therapy* (1915).

The *Text-book of Osteopathy* illustrated manipulation of the spine, shoulder, and back, and rotation of the leg and thigh, plus stretching and massage. Components of

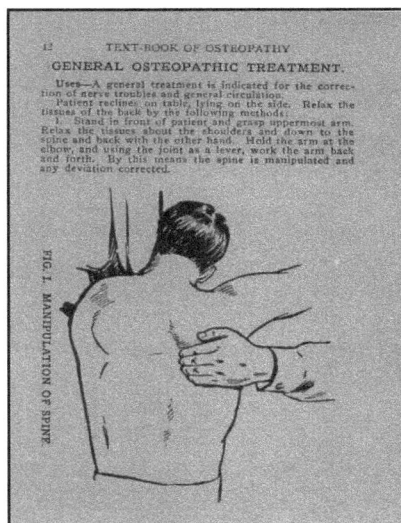

Text-Book of Osteopathy (1910) **American College of Mechano-Therapy (Chicago)** (Courtesy of the National Archives – Digital collection public domain)

chiropractic and zone therapy too. Lizzie and her father were so impressed with these treatments that she enrolled in the one-year course and received a scholarship on March 3, 1909.

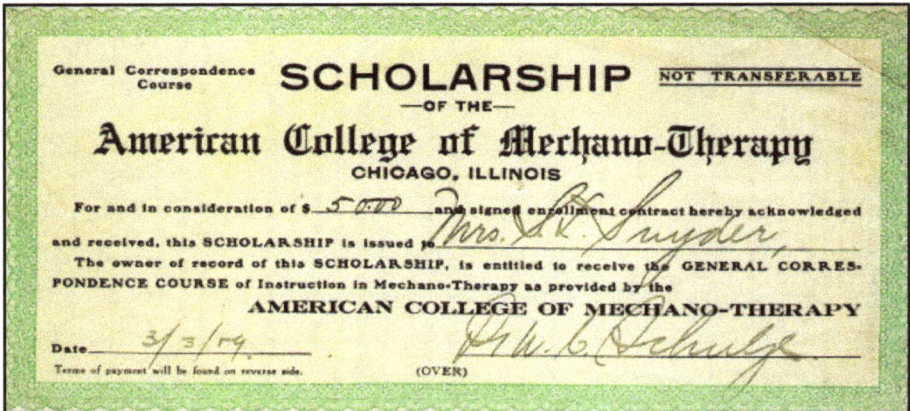

AMERICAN COLLEGE OF MECHANO-THERAPY SCHOLARSHIP
(Author's collection)

The remodel of Lizzie's home had also begun. The front door was relocated to the far left, a covered porch and planked walkway added, and the interior was restructured with a parlor that served as the reception and waiting area. A portion of the living quarters were sectioned off into treatment rooms.

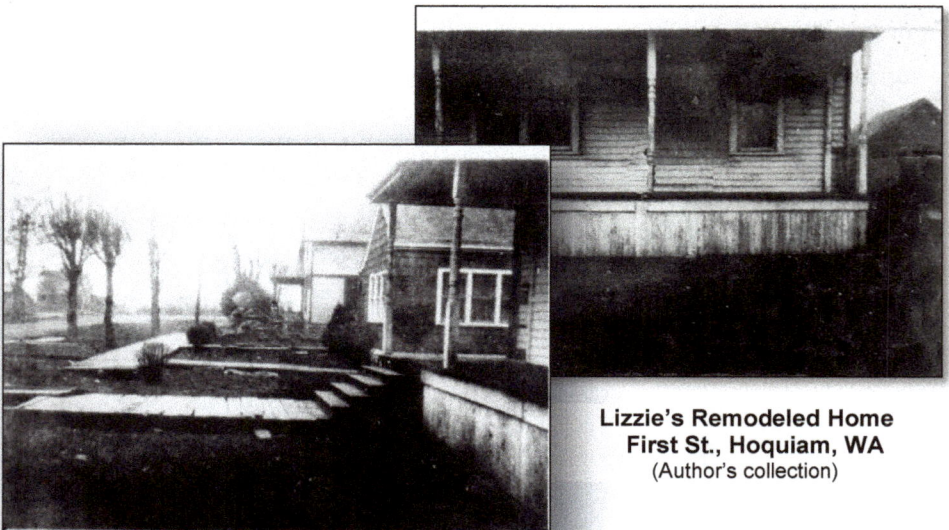

**Lizzie's Remodeled Home
First St., Hoquiam, WA**
(Author's collection)

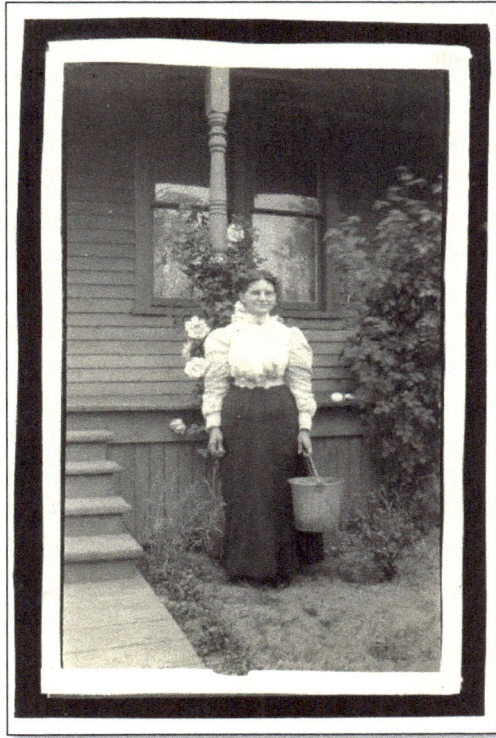

Lizzie in front of remodeled home

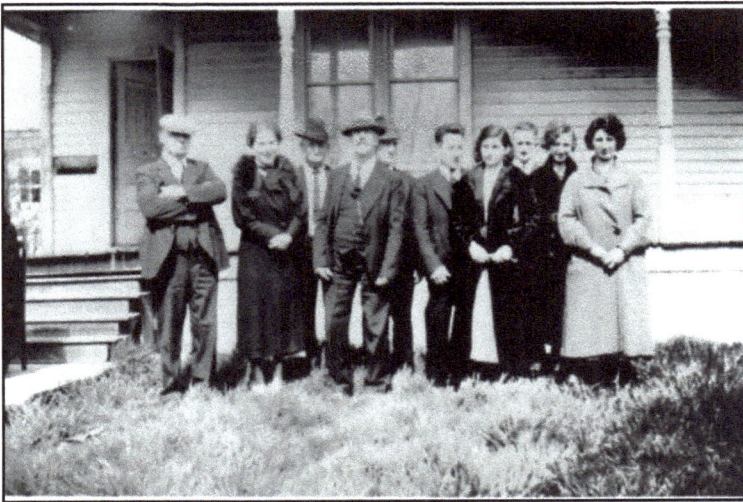

Family and friends in front of Lizzie's home (1920s)
(All photos: Author's collection)

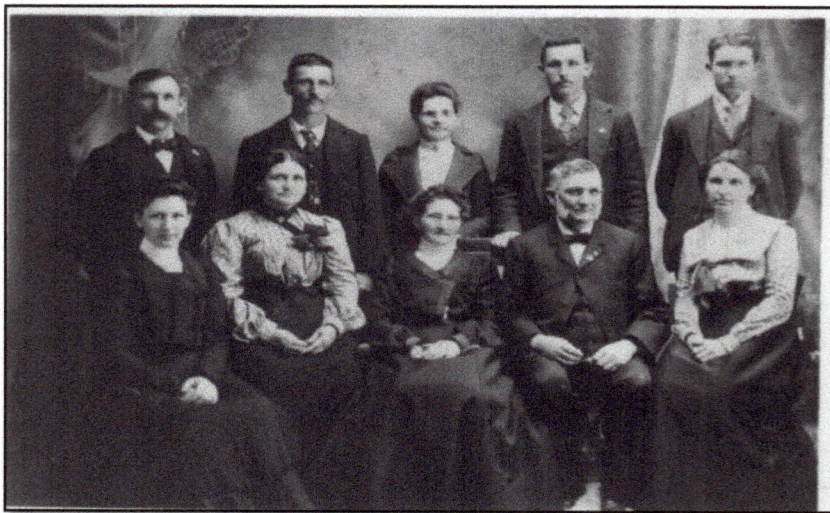

Wilson Family Photo, 1909
(Author's collection)

Back L to R: Jackson (A.J.), Charles, **Lizzie**, Fred, Frank
Front L to R: Lulu, Catherine, Mother, Father, Josephine

1910 Postcard to Mrs. W.B. Wilson (Mary)
1315 Riverside, Hoquiam, WA
(Author's collection)

7
ON HER OWN

ONE CAN IMAGINE the family's distress when they heard that Father was hurt, with a brief explanation that he fell out of bed. The doctor had been summoned, but the only answer was to wait. For three days Lizzie tried different therapies. On January 13, 1910, W.B. Wilson passed away. His death certificate stated: "Patient pitched out of bed at night onto his forehead—accidental fall. Resultant: inflammation of forehead and face."

Through the years, Lizzie had stepped in for her father, such as the period when he had traveled to Tacoma, so she was accustomed to treating patients on her own, but not without his guidance. She continued treating, but at a slower pace. She also completed her Mechano-Therapy studies and on February 9, 1911, received her diploma as Professor S.L. Snyder, Doctor of Mechano-Therapy.

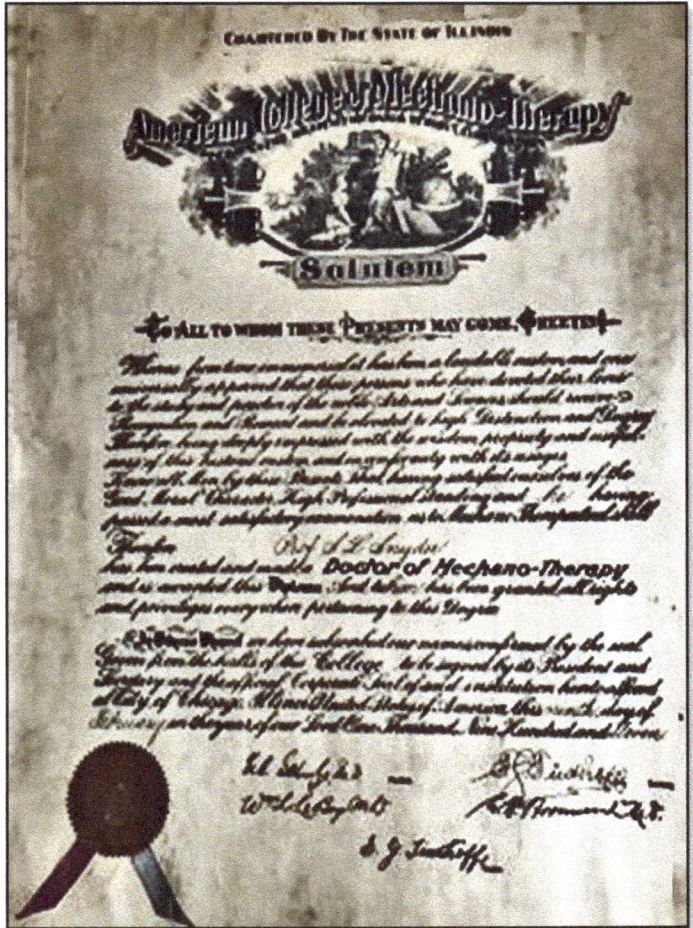

**FEB 9, 1911
PROF. S.L. SNYDER
MECHANO-THERAPY
DIPLOMA**
(Author's collection)

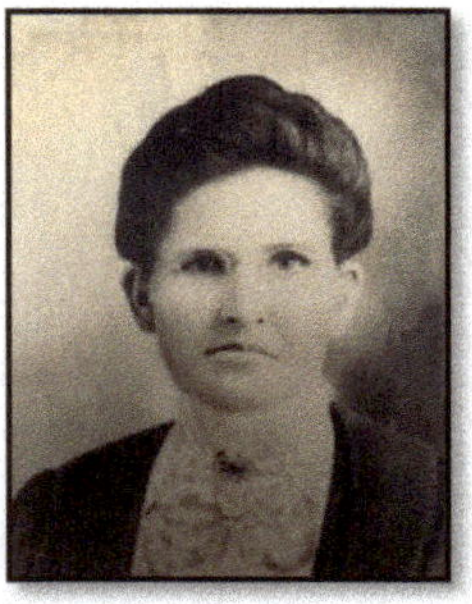

Lizzie 1911
(Age 48)

With a diploma of her own, Lizzie began expanding her practice. On May 1911, she teamed up with a traveling healer, Dr. Jefferson. Prior to arriving in Aberdeen, he placed an ad for an assistant. Lizzie promptly replied and sponsored his setup at a local Aberdeen hotel. On June 11, 1911, he placed an advertisement in the *Washingtonian,* the local newspaper, listing the "Snyder Hotel, 1934 Heron Street, Aberdeen" as his headquarters. Lizzie quickly corrected the error, marking up his original advertisement for reprint to state: "His work carried on at headquarters by his assistant, S.L. Snyder, First Str, Hoquiam, Wash."

JUNE 11, 1911

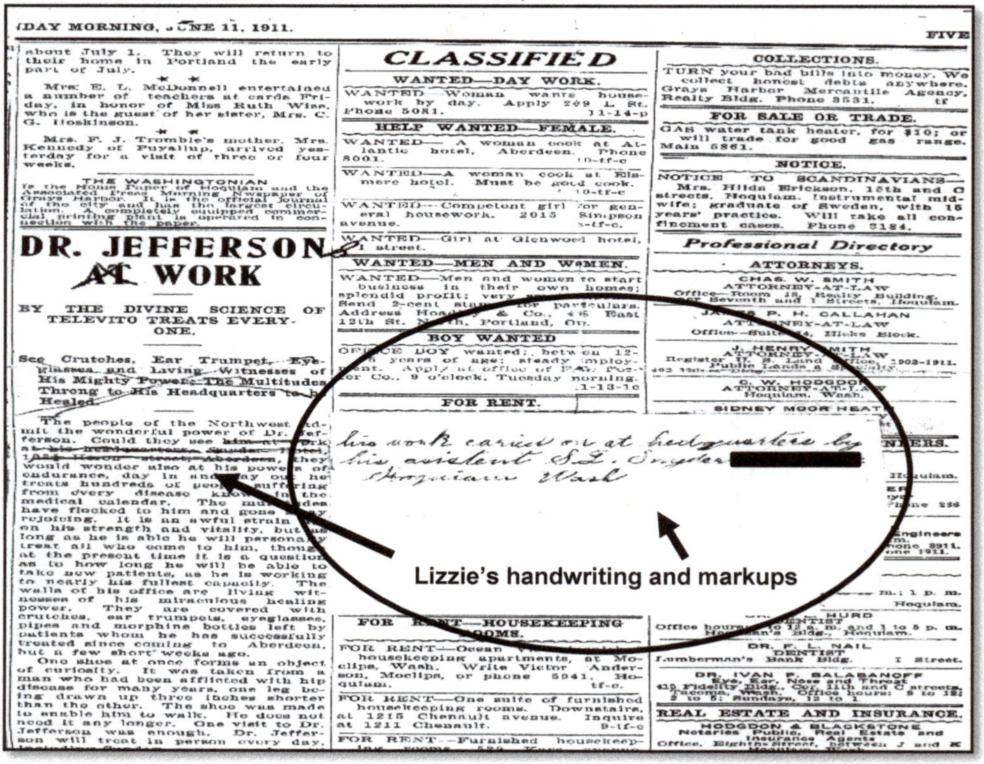

DR. JEFFERSON'S ORIGINAL AD WITH LIZZIE'S MARKUPS
(Author's collection)

Based on his next ad, it appears that Dr. Jefferson was lending his credentials to Lizzie and she was providing use of her home as his headquarters. More than likely, a business arrangement was drawn up of shared revenue for new patients for an extended period. The crux of his healing message was the "Divine Science of Televito," which followed the New Thought format, but had samplings of the Weltmer methods too, such as Absent Treatments.

In the heading of the ad, Lizzie is referenced as his student and appointed as his assistant. Her home address is listed as his headquarters.

Dr. Jefferson's
Second Ad. Excerpt.
Est. Date (June 20, 1911)

The people of the Northwest admit the wonderful power of Dr. Jefferson. Could they see the work at his headquarters, "S.L. Snyder, First Street, Hoquiam." They would wonder also at his powers of endurance, day in and day out, he treats hundreds of people suffering from every disease known in the medical calendar.

(Author's collection)

DR. JEFFERSON'S WORK

BY THE DIVINE SCIENCE OF TELEVITO TREATS.

By His Student Appointed As His Assistant. Witnesses of His Mighty Power; The Multitude Throng to His Headquarters to be Healed.

The people of the Northwest admit the wonderful power of Dr. Jefferson. Could they see the work at his headquarters. S. L. Snyder, street Hoquiam. They would wonder also at his powers of endurance day in and day out he treats hundreds of people suffering from every disease known in the medical calendar. He does this freely, his sole object seeming to be to heal all he can. The multitudes have flocked to him and gone away rejoicing. It is an awful strain upon his strength and vitality, but as long as he is able he will personally treat all who come to him.

The mail received by him is larger than ever and constantly increasing, while a large corps of assistants are necessary to handle part of his practice. Each letter receives his personal attention and is promptly answered. Many communications have been received where the parties seem loth to give him their confidence; we would say do not be afraid to write fully and freely, it will be promptly answered and in the strictest confidence. He must thoroughly understand your needs before being enabled to treat you as successfully as he would desire. His power can be transmitted as effectively by his absence method as by the personal treatments. We wish to append many testimonials of people who have been completely restored to health through this method. These people can each one be addressed for proof of these statements. Mrs. C. De Lorme, 1981 Main street, Hartford, Conn., cured of nerve and heart trouble in six treatments. Mrs. Amelia K. Green of Honolulu was cured by fifteen absent treatments of nervous prostration and rheumatism. Healer Jefferson is treating by the absent method several patients there for leprosy with successful results. Miss Frances Howell of Concord, N. H., had a large tumor of three years' growth. Many physicians whom she consulted told her nothing but a surgical operation could remove it. She was cured after twenty-two treatments and is now perfectly healthy. Mrs. W. W. Miller of Marblehead, Mass., was subject for years to chronic headaches which had resulted in the partial paralysis of the optic nerve. She was completely cured by twenty-five absent treatments. A child of fourteen from Quebec, who had suffered for years from a com-

As his assistant, Lizzie provided Absent Treatments under Dr. Jefferson's name. Excerpts from his second ad, June 20, 1911, stated:

- *The mail received by him is larger than ever and constantly increasing, while a large corps of assistants are necessary to handle part of his practice.*
- *We would say do not be afraid to write fully and freely, it will be promptly answered and in the strictest confidence.*
- *Mrs. Amelia K. Green of Honolulu was cured by fifteen absent treatments of nervous prostration and rheumatism.*

Excerpt from his first ad, June 11, 1911, which Lizzie had corrected and reprinted in the newspaper:

The walls of his office are living witnesses of his miraculous healing power. They are covered with crutches, ear trumpets, eyeglasses, pipes, and morphine bottles left by patients whom he has successfully treated since coming to Aberdeen, but a few short weeks ago.

Several of the methods listed in his ads, such as testimonials both by him and his patients, point to Dr. Jefferson as one of the earlier healers from the same era as Lizzie's father and reveal the Weltmer influence. His reference, however, to "The Divine Science of Televito" suggest that he didn't follow the Weltmer doctrine that the power was all in the Creator, instead he leaned toward New Thought.

Many New Thought members read *Weltmer's Magazine* and attended the New Thought Convention sponsored by Weltmer, but they believed that a higher power pervaded all existence and that individuals could create their own reality via affirmations, meditation, and prayer. The Church of Divine Science was one of several that practiced this theory. It is also noted that Weltmer referred to his healers as professors, not doctors. In fact, Weltmer recognized the need for medical care when other options failed.[1] New Thought believed the opposite.

DR. JEFFERSON DISAPPEARED as quickly as he had arrived, and when Lizzie placed her own ad in the newspaper, there was no mention of him. She did follow his format by referencing the Power of Televito. One of her artifacts was a 1907 book by William Walker Atkinson. Atkinson was the editor of *New Thought* magazine and had authored over one-hundred books on related topics, so she was open to both views. Even though Lizzie's ad emphasized the Divine Science of Televito, most of her training had been Weltmer and she never deviated from his core teachings or beliefs. Her advertisements also included Absent Treatments, a Weltmer trademark.

Excerpt from Lizzie's September 1911 newspaper ad:

This power can be transmitted as effectively by the absent method as by the personal treatment. Only write plainly and fully the details of your case as there must be a thorough understanding of each case to treat successfully. Every inquiry will be answered promptly and held in strictest confidence.

Mental Magic, Atkinson's 300-page lesson book, addressed underlying principles of the why's and how's that personal influence and personal magnetism operated.

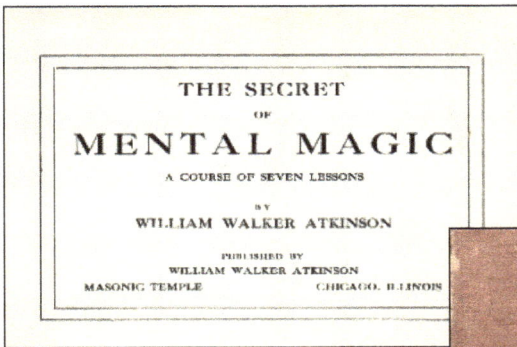

MENTAL MAGIC
S.L. Snyder artifact
(Author's collection)

Another book in Lizzie's possession was *Regeneration*, Weltmer's 1908 copyrighted edition. Various pages were bookmarked and underlined. One that was earmarked by Lizzie was the section on "Courage." One might think after her father's death, she was searching for insight and guidance. Excerpt from *Regeneration*:

> *Courage is not a thing which can be acquired by long years of practice.*
> *YOU CAN ACQUIRE IT IN A MOMENT. To be courageous you*
> *need not have a strong, robust body. You do not need to have your*
> *nervous system in perfect repair to be a brave man or woman, but you*
> *do need to have a determination to accomplish some particular purpose*
> *in life, no matter what it costs. Courage is that impulse which comes into*
> *a human soul and makes it put everything in balance; no matter what the*
> *result—follow the chosen course—the goal of which is mastery.*[2]

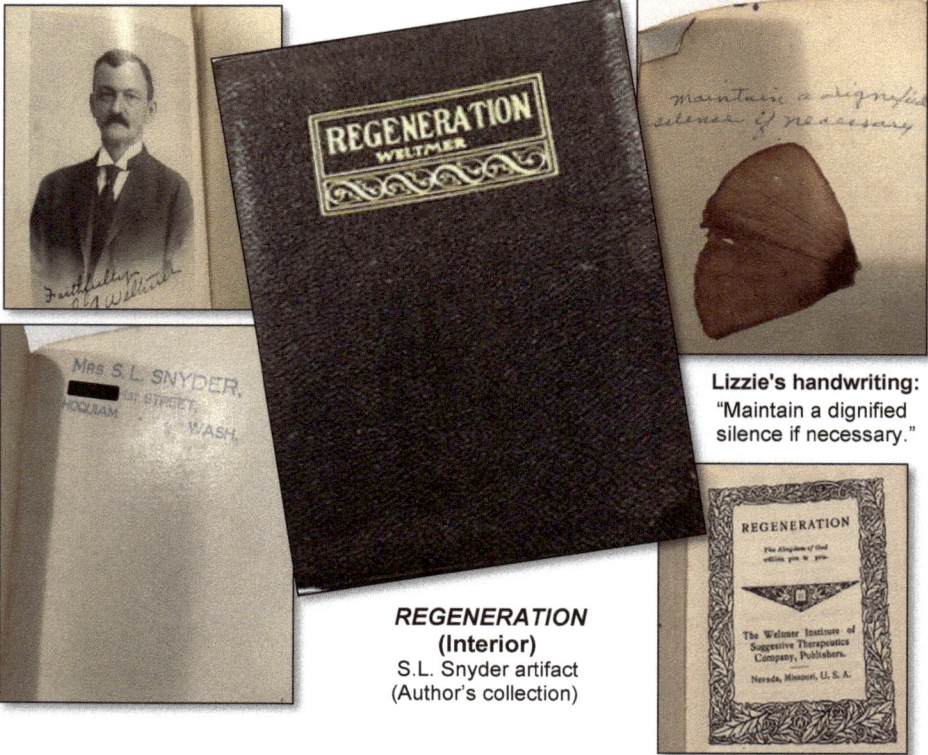

Lizzie's handwriting:
"Maintain a dignified silence if necessary."

REGENERATION
(Interior)
S.L. Snyder artifact
(Author's collection)

SEPTEMBER, 1911

LIZZIE'S *WASHINGTONIAN* NEWSPAPER AD
(Sept 1911)
(Author's collection)

Excerpt from Lizzie's September 1911 ad:

Only three cents per mile. Out of town folks can come and see her. For $3, the price of an ordinary doctor's examination, you can travel 100 miles and get the advice free. It will pay you to come 2,000 miles to be treated by the Divine Science of Televito.

In addition to an advertising strategy, listing the Divine Science of Televito offered an element of mystery. Most who sought unorthodox healers were seeking new answers where the traditional treatments and medicines had failed.

Excerpt from Lizzie's September 1911 ad:

The cured, satisfied patients dismissed, who before coming to her for treatment, had become almost physical and mental wrecks, are the best evidence that could be given as the power of Televito. The many sufferers who come to her from friends of theirs who have tried the science, is a proof of the power.

The majority of Lizzie's patients were women from the Victorian era who were not comfortable talking to a male doctor. Weltmer stressed the following protocol in his teachings: "When treating a woman, the male practitioner should require the attendance of a relative or a nurse."

John Snyder's assessment of Lizzie in his 1894 letter provides insight of her character: "Your nature is sympathetic, love of nature, of good ideas, of duty. The gift of the power of authority in you is more than an average, well qualified to make all happy that is around you, your council is good and your decision is good."

Based in his evaluation, Lizzie possessed the traits of a compassionate and competent person who could be trusted to listen, guide, and council to the best of her ability. The testimonial from the gentleman in her ad, who lived in Elma approximately forty-five minutes from Lizzie's practice, offered a view of his condition, which was partially attributed to bad habits. With Lizzie's treatments, it appears that his disorders reversed before they became serious ailments.

Excerpt from Lizzie's September 1911 ad (gentleman's testimonial):

Elma, Wash., August 30, 1911.
Dear Madam of Divinity—I do not know what to tell you, only that I am
well and that I am thankful.

These are the remarks of a party after three weeks treatment for heart
failure, stomach trouble, constipation, and excessive tobacco chewing.
Before treatment he had to carry around with him a bottle of whisky to
revive him when he would swoon away and morphine pills to stop the
pain.

The course of his treatment would have included Weltmer's "Laying on of Hands" combined with the "Power of Suggestion and Prayer." Mechano-Therapy may have also been used and the replacement of the tobacco, whisky, and morphine with Lizzie's herbal remedies would have also helped.

AFTER THE September 1911 newspaper ad, there is no evidence that Lizzie continued advertising in the newspaper. She went back to her father's format of word of mouth and handing out calling cards. She also belonged to several organizations. One was the Hoquiam W.C.T.U. (Woman's Christian Temperance Union). From her marriage to Hanson, she knew firsthand the demons of those who drank. The purpose of the W.C.T.U. was for a sober and pure world through abstinence and Christianity. They also supported community and missionary causes, and later, the Women's Suffrage movement.

Excerpt from *School Days' 1900,* Page 9, by Clara Knack Dooley describes the Hoquiam W.C.T.U:

They had a parade in the morning of the Fourth of July, and we liked to
watch it. The only part I remember now of the parade was the part of the
W.C.T.U. (The Women's [sic] Christian Temperance Union) made up
of women in their long black skirts and white blouses (or rather shirt
waists) most of them wearing a little black bow membership pin, with
stern expressions on their faces, marching along in military style. I always
think of one woman who looked as if she could bite nails in two. [3]

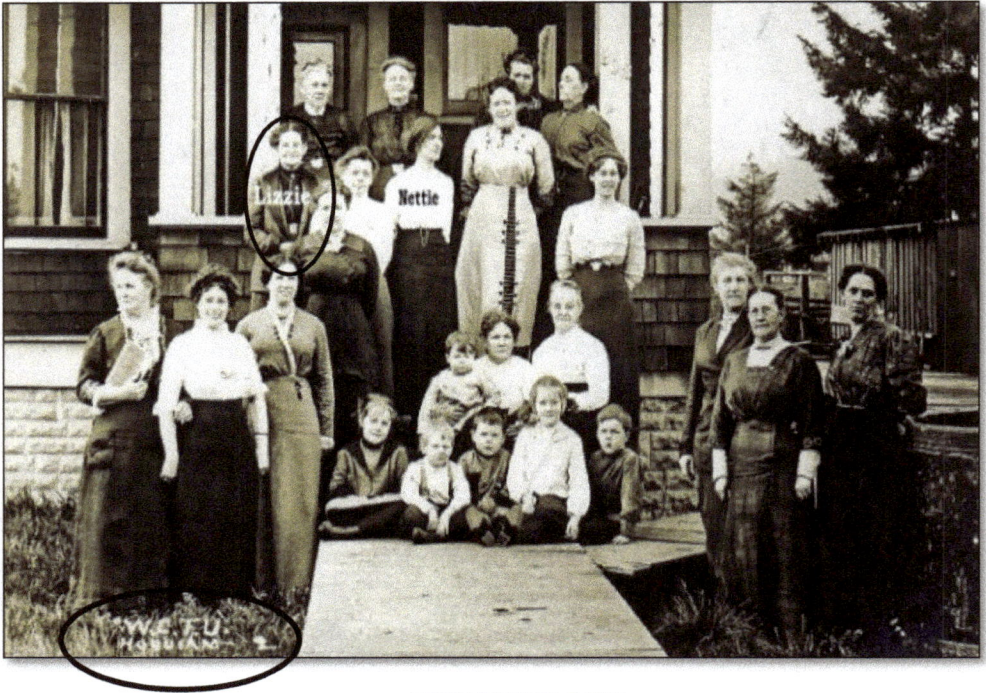

HOQUIAM W.C.T.U.
Great-Grandmother's Lizzie Snyder & Nettie Connell Taylor
(Author's collection)

Lizzie attended events with husband, John, who was a city councilman, a member of various committees and clubs, and a candidate for constable. John's community work and high standing brought creditability to Lizzie's healing practice.

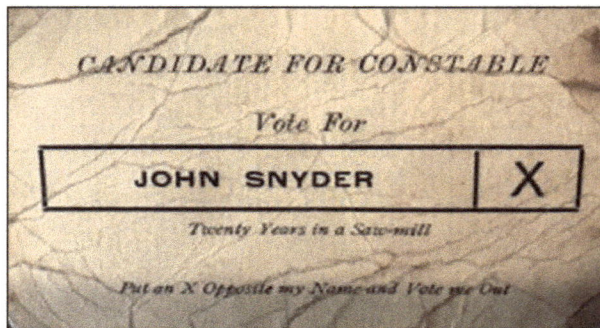

(Author's collection)

**1909 & 1910
Hoquiam City Council
Booklet**
(Author's collection)

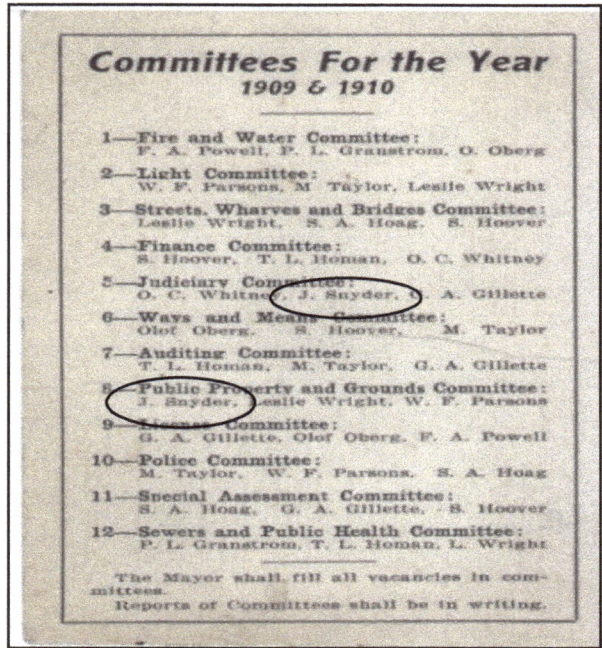

**Committees For the Year
1909 & 1910**

1—Fire and Water Committee:
F. A. Powell, P. L. Granstrom, O. Oberg

2—Light Committee:
W. F. Parsons, M. Taylor, Leslie Wright

3—Streets, Wharves and Bridges Committee:
Leslie Wright, S. A. Hoag, S. Hoover

4—Finance Committee:
S. Hoover, T. L. Homan, O. C. Whitney

5—Judiciary Committee:
O. C. Whitney, J. Snyder, G. A. Gillette

6—Ways and Means Committee:
Olof Oberg, S. Hoover, M. Taylor

7—Auditing Committee:
T. L. Homan, M. Taylor, G. A. Gillette

8—Public Property and Grounds Committee:
J. Snyder, Leslie Wright, W. F. Parsons

9—License Committee:
G. A. Gillette, Olof Oberg, F. A. Powell

10—Police Committee:
M. Taylor, W. F. Parsons, S. A. Hoag

11—Special Assessment Committee:
S. A. Hoag, G. A. Gillette, S. Hoover

12—Sewers and Public Health Committee:
P. L. Granstrom, T. L. Homan, L. Wright

The Mayor shall fill all vacancies in committees.
Reports of Committees shall be in writing.

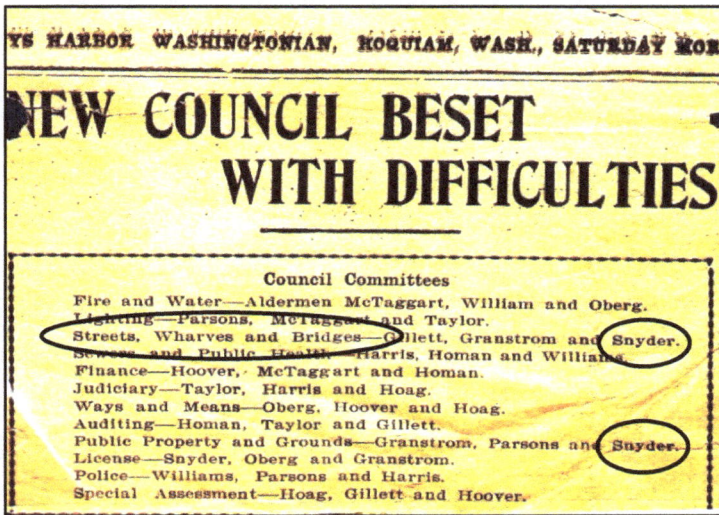

GRAYS HARBOR WASHINGTONIAN, HOQUIAM, WASH., SATURDAY MORNING

NEW COUNCIL BESET WITH DIFFICULTIES

Council Committees

Fire and Water—Aldermen McTaggart, William and Oberg.
Lighting—Parsons, McTaggart and Taylor.
Streets, Wharves and Bridges—Gillett, Granstrom and Snyder.
Sewers and Public Health—Harris, Homan and Williams.
Finance—Hoover, McTaggart and Homan.
Judiciary—Taylor, Harris and Hoag.
Ways and Means—Oberg, Hoover and Hoag.
Auditing—Homan, Taylor and Gillett.
Public Property and Grounds—Granstrom, Parsons and Snyder.
License—Snyder, Oberg and Granstrom.
Police—Williams, Parsons and Harris.
Special Assessment—Hoag, Gillett and Hoover.

1910 *WASHINGTONIAN* NEWSPAPER
(Author's collection)

While serving on the Streets, Wharves, and Bridges' committee, John received a postcard, postmarked from Egypt, from George H. Emerson, one of the founding fathers of Hoquiam and of the Northwestern Lumber Company.

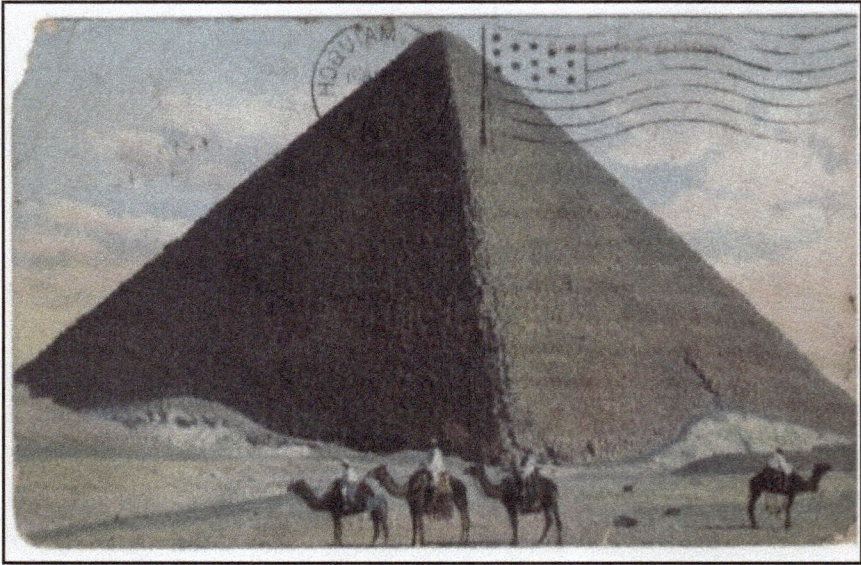

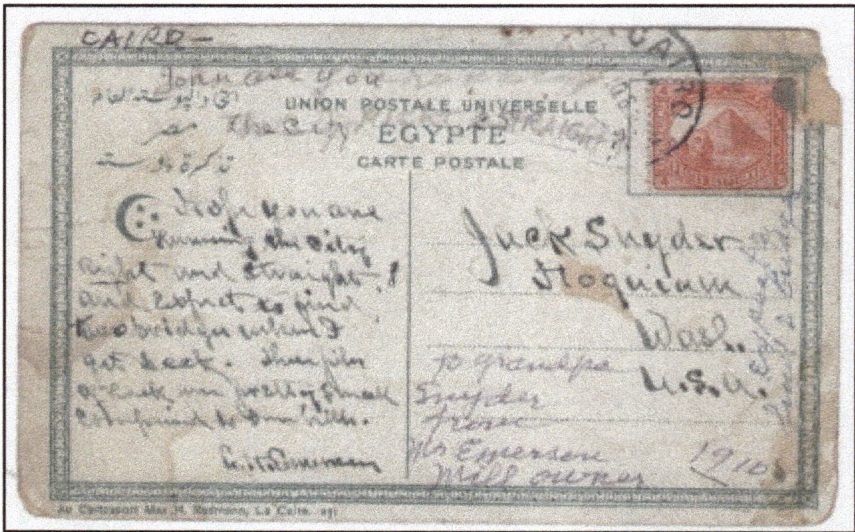

GEORGE EMERSON POSTCARD (1910)
Cairo, Egypt
(Author's collection)

Excerpt: "John, you are running the city right and straight! And expect to find two bridges when I get back." Geo. H. Emerson.

8
NEW HORIZONS

BY 1915 LIZZIE'S LIFE had shifted. Lizzie's mother had passed away the prior year and Mr. Lee years before. Her youngest children: Jessie was married with a baby on the way, Lincoln off working, and Florence, seventeen, in her final year of high school. Lizzie, approaching fifty-two, had been running her healing practice for almost five years. When she saw the four-year-college advertisement in *Weltmer's Magazine*, she was redirected onto a new path.

ESTABLISHED FEBRUARY 15, 1897

We Have Builded Our Reputation upon the Cures of "Hopeless" Cases

SCHOOL ════════ SANITARIUM

In the School we give a Four Year Course of personal instruction, comprising twenty-four months' attendance in classes, preceded by 180 hours of home study, from text books we furnish to all students without additional charge.

The Weltmer Institute is the parent school of Weltmerism, Magnetic Healing, Laying on of Hands, Mental Science and the other drugless methods which may be included under broad general head of Suggestive Therapeutics.

The Weltmer Institute has a well-organized faculty which has been working together for fifteen years, and lately we have made several excellent additions, We teach the subject together with corrollary branches necessary to the professional and financial success of the graduate, in a thorough and systematic manner.

Special advantages to Students enrolling, for March classes, before February 15, 1915.

17th ANNUAL CATALOG, WILL BE SENT POSTPAID—GRATIS UPON REQUEST

CUT ON THIS LINE—NOW

The Sanitarium connected with the Weltmer School is equipped with every modern facility.

Patients rooms have electric light, steam heat, hot and cold water, roomy clothes closet, good ventilation.

We have regular physicians constantly employed in the Sanitarium and School; however, nearly all cases are cured without the use of drugs or surgery. Patients attending our Sanitarium receive benefits of every safe, sane and effective method of cure, and for one fee, which is less than the charge made at most sanitarium for the one particular method which happens to be the fad of the physician in charge.

All Year Health Resort, Nevada, Mo., U.S.A.

POST CARD

Place Stamp Here

Weltmer Institute of Suggestotherapy,

206 SOUTH ASH STREET

Nevada, Mo.,

U.S.A.

The Weltmer Institute has in 17 years pleased 262,000 patrons from all parts of the world—has builded its reputation upon the cures of "Hopeless" cases—in a beautiful city of 10,000 population—Park with lake and three mineral wells—Ozark climate—altitude 1100 feet—expenses very moderate. Particulars free, upon request.

WELTMER INSTITUTE FOUR-YEAR AD
The State Historical Society of Missouri (SHSMO) Artifact
(Courtesy of the Bushwhacker Museum, Nevada, Mo.)

THE CLINICAL COURSE for a degree comprised of four terms, six months each, preceded by 180 hours of preparatory study. Enrollment period was the week prior to the first week of March and September of each year. Due to her age and experience, Lizzie more than likely didn't have to meet the standard enrollment requirements, such as proof of an eighth-grade education in a public school, soon to be changed to a four-year high school prerequisite, and a certificate of good moral character signed by two professional or business men from the student's community.

Tuition for the four-year course including the $50 preparatory study was $450, but reduced to $425 if paid in full. The student could also pay the $100 yearly tuition by year, which would have been the path Lizzie would have chosen. The payment included tuition, text books, diploma, dissection material, and all laboratory charges excluding any broken or destroyed apparatus by the student. Room, board, and laundry were an extra expense and ranged from $75 to $260 per year, depending on the accommodations.

For one year of expenses, Lizzie would have needed approximately $650 [p] to cover the school costs, room and board, train passage, plus incidentals. In 1915, Lizzie had some money saved from her practice in her S.L. Snyder savings, but nothing near the $650 needed.

Based on John's savings in 1889, some of it from inheritance, it is believed that he had at least $500 remaining and that Lizzie's eldest children, Mary Belle, William, and Lester also contributed.

No. 960

The Bank of Hoquiam
HOQUIAM, WASH.

SAVINGS DEPARTMENT

BANKING HOURS
9 A.M. TO 3 P.M.

S.L. Snyder

This Book must be presented when money is deposited or withdrawn.

**S.L. Snyder &
John Snyder's
Separate Savings
Accounts**
(Author's collection)

**Year 1889, John's balance
after withdraws = $1,550**

---

[p] About $18,000 in today's money.

During the summers, Mary Belle and sea-captain husband, Fred Cline, and family lived aboard their steamboat, the *Irene.* During fishing season, they trolled the Columbia River for Royal Chinook salmon and averaged $200 [q] or more per week. William and Lester, plus other family members often joined them to earn extra money.

AS JULY 1916 APPROACHED, Lizzie had completed the 180-hours of preparatory home study, placed her healing practice on hiatus, and with the birth of Jessie's daughter, Lizzie became a grandmother for the fifth time. She had also secured lodging at a boarding house near the institute and paid in advance for one year of courses.

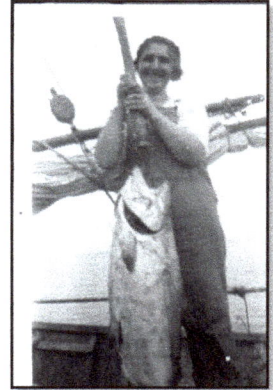

Florence Snyder (17)
50lb+ salmon
on the *Irene*

The day of departure, John, Lincoln, and Florence were on the platform as she boarded the train. The trip would have been at least a four-to-five-day journey. She more than likely purchased a second-class ticket with upholstered seats and paid extra for a sleeping berth.

Based on a 1914 reply received from Aunt Mattie about Lizzie's mother, Mary Wilson's passing, shows that Lizzie communicated with her aunt on important subjects and would have scheduled a visit to Nebraska

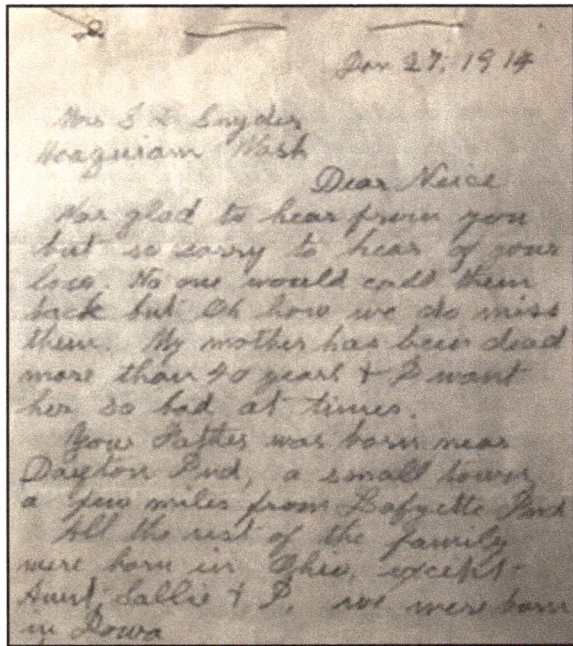

1914 Letter from Aunt Mattie
(Author's collection)

---

[q] About $5,500 in today's money.

on her way to the Weltmer Institute. A 1936 letter from Mattie's daughter to Florence Snyder substantiates that visit.

Excerpt of May 12, 1936 letter:

I met your mother (Lizzie) *just once, the short time she visited here when she was back here on a trip, so that Ma* (Mattie) *was much better acquainted with her than I. Ma leaves all the writing to me, as all she can manage to do is sign her name.*

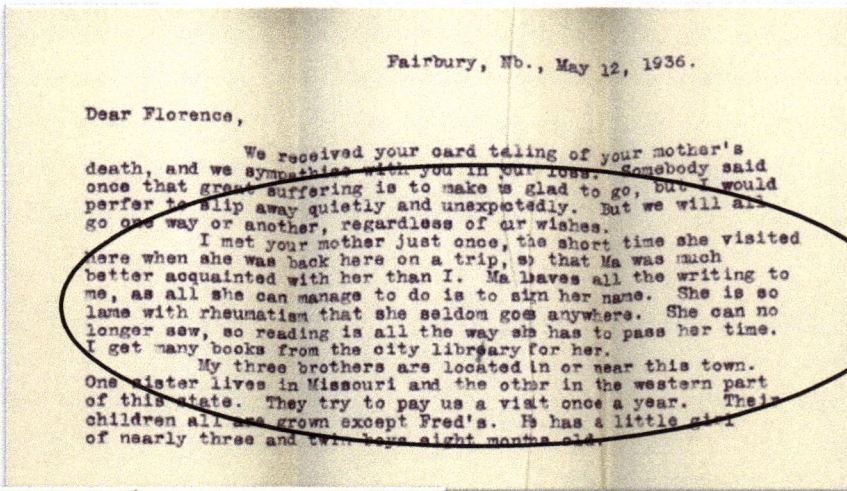

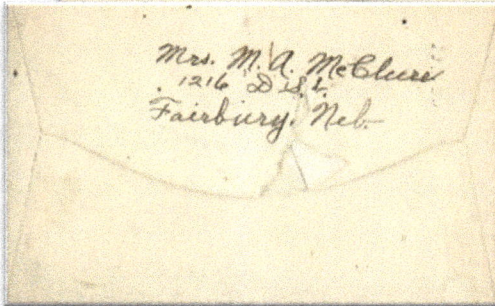

1936 Letter from Mattie's Daughter
(Author's collection)

It had been forty-six years, since 1870, that Lizzie and Mattie had seen one another. Lizzie was eight, and Mattie, a young bride in her early twenties. They had all been living in Holt, Missouri. Mattie's new husband, Mordecai McClure, was working with Lizzie's father in the sawmill. Before Lizzie had eye surgery, Mattie and Mordecai relocated to Nebraska, so she never saw Lizzie regain her sight. One can only imagine their reunion and Mattie's delight to be seeing Lizzie again. After the visit, Lizzie continued on for another fifteen hours or so to the Weltmer Institute in Nevada, Missouri.

WHEN LIZZIE'S FATHER ATTENDED the institute in 1900, it was called "S.A. Weltmer School of Healing." In March 1906, it had rechartered and was renamed "Weltmer Institute of Suggestive Therapeutics." Suggestive Therapeutics, also referred to as Science of Healing, was based on philosophical and biological considerations. The theory was that the body could manufacture serums and secretions for its own repair and growth, and when properly directed and given a chance, could achieve this goal. It was through thoughts that the mind healed the body, and that these thoughts were determined by suggestions received from the environment. [1] The Suggestive Therapist, through his suggestions, would synchronize the thoughts through oral and manual suggestions, many times in combination.

With oral suggestions, the therapist would speak into the deeper mind of the patient, past the conscious mind and into the healing one. Manual suggestions were performed through the "Laying on of Hands," and viewed by Weltmer as the most beneficial. He believed that the healing power though the hands influenced powerful suggestions to the sensory nerves and directly to the healing mind. [2] So, when Lizzie attended, not only had the institute restructured its name, but its curriculum as well.

> Through the thoughts it forms, the mind controls (heals) the body. Thoughts are largely determined by suggestions received from environment. The Suggestive Therapist determines by means of his suggestions what thoughts shall act upon the body.

SUGGESTIVE THERAPIST
DESCRIPTION
Back of Lizzie's Membership Card
(Author's collection)

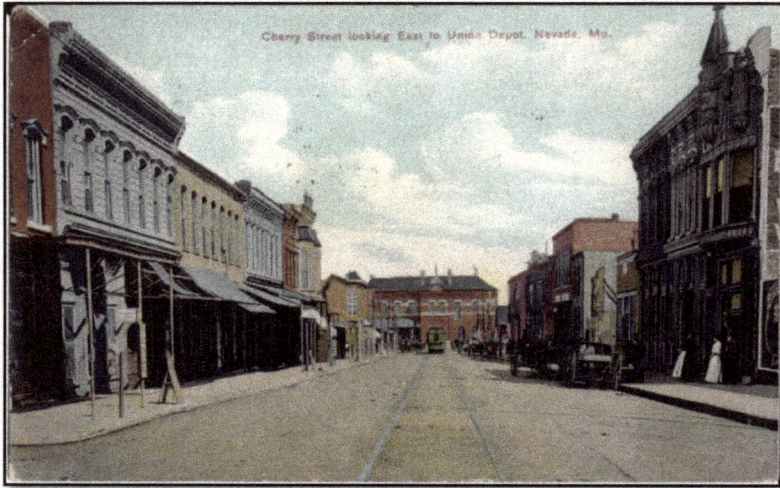

CHERRY STREET, Nevada, Missouri
Looking toward Union Depot
(Courtesy of the Bushwhacker Museum, Nevada, Mo.)

AS THE TRAIN pulled into the Nevada station, Lizzie's father had to be in her thoughts. He had arrived sixteen years prior for treatment and left as Professor W.B. Wilson, magnetic healer. Back then, students were transported to the institute by horse and buggy. Now, they were advised to follow the electric railway line nine blocks west and one block south. Another option was to request an identification badge beforehand and to be met by an agent with a free carriage ride to the institute. [3]

All new students were instructed to report directly to the general office before making any arrangements. Even though Lizzie had secured her own lodging and selected the courses she wanted to attend, it may have been changed once she arrived at the facility. Furnished rooms, requiring light housekeeping, were offered for $9 to $20[r] per month. Cottages were also available at $2 to $8 per month, but no meals and some were unfurnished.

Lizzie stayed at a boardinghouse close to the institute with modest rates. Except for the light housekeeping as part of their room and board, students were not allowed to work. All monies for expenses had to be available before the start of each quarter.

---

[r] $9 is about $247 in today's money. $20 is about $549.

FOR PERMANENT HEALTH

Fresh Air—Pure Water—Wholesome Food—Relaxation and Sleep—Outdoor Exercise—Cleanliness of Mind and Body—Regular Habits—Useful Work—Cheerful Thoughts, will, when taken in proper portions and utilized under the direction of a constructive mental attitude, make and keep you well; and bring you the greatest mental and physical efficiency.

If you are sick it is because you have been taking too much of one and not enough of the others, or, you have taken all of some and none of the others.

We enable you to regain your health and teach you how to keep it.

EXPENSES AT NEVADA, MISSOURI

PATIENT'S DEPARTMENT

ROOM, MEALS AND TREATMENT IN SANITARIUM—$19.50 to $50.00 per week. ROOM IN ANNEX—With meals and treatment in Sanitarium, $17.50 to $21.50 per week.

MEAL TICKET IN SANITARIUM—$4.00 per week. (Extra charge for a la carte service).

14 ROOMS at $1.00 per day each for two occupants or $1.50 per day for one occupant.

15 ROOMS with access to private bath and toilet at $1.50 to $3.50 per day.

32 Rooms with running water, steam heat, electric light and modern conveniences.

ALL RATES based on American plan but a la carte service in dining room may be secured by special arrangement.

REGULAR TREATMENT UNDER DIRECTION OF SANITARIUM PHYSICIAN—$12.50 (minimum) per week of six treatments.

All departments of the Weltmer Institute are under the supervision of Prof. Sidney A. Weltmer, its founder and President. However, he treats regularly only a limited number of cases. The charge in such cases is $25.00 (minimum) for five treatments per week.

BATH—All kinds of bath and massage, 25 cents to $2.50.

RAILROAD RATES—Patients who can receive a cure in less than 90 days should secure special railroad rates, which are now in effect to Nevada, from many parts of the country.—Write us for particulars.

STUDENT'S DEPARTMENT

FOUR YEAR COLLEGIATE COURSE—Conferring Diploma and Degree of D. S. T. $450.00, minus all former payments for text books, Correspondence Courses or short courses. Enrollments are now being accepted for the first year class opening Sept. 1st, 1913.

SHORT COURSE IN ESSENTIALS OF SUGGESTIVE THERAPEUTICS—Conferring DIPLOMA giving credit for all work completed and title S. T.

THE LAST SHORT COURSE BEGINS MAY 5TH, 1913, AND ENDS AUGUST 16TH, 1913.

Tuition, including Complete Correspondence Course and text books to the value of $100.00—is $150.00. No extra charge for apparatus or dissection.

COMPLETE CORRESPONDENCE COURSE IN SUGGESTIVE THERAPEUTICS AND APPLIED PSYCHOLOGY—with privilege of personal instruction and conferring CERTIFICATE OF GRADUATION is $85.00 cash or $100.00 on easy payments.

Students can take furnished rooms and live in Nevada (at light housekeeping), for $5.00 to $20.00 per month.

They can get cottages (sometimes furnished) for $2.00 to $5.00 per room per month, or they can get any other accommodations within reasonable prices.

Students and patients will find all manner of seasonable amusements at Nevada; good horses for riding and driving; good roads for automobiling; also tennis, baseball, basket-ball, canoeing, et cetera. At Radio Springs and Park there are most beautiful surroundings for a day in the open. In this remarkable park are found three mineral springs of pure and curative water. These springs fill two large lakes with fresh water, making an excellent place for bathing, rowing and fishing, all of which are enjoyed by thousands every year.

Write us for IDENTIFICATION BADGE, and an agent of the Weltmer Institute with FREE CARRIAGE will meet you at the train and assist with invalids and baggage, and bring you to the Sanitarium or find suitable accommodations.

Railway connections to Nevada are convenient from all directions. We have through trains from almost all near-by railway centers. You can wire us from any near-by railway center and our station agent will meet you at the depot without fail.

Authorized by the Officers and Faculty of the Weltmer Institute of Suggestive Therapeutics Company, 1913-14. Ben T. Taylor, M. D., House Physician.

EXPENSES AT NEVADA, MISSOURI
The State Historical Society of Missouri (SHSMO) Artifact
(Courtesy of the Bushwhacker Museum, Nevada, Mo.)

Lizzie's experience as an osteopath qualified her for the "advanced-standing" option, available to registered medical doctors, osteopaths, and graduates from other recognized osteopathic or medical colleges. Once proper credentials were received: a recent photograph and subscription for the 180-hour preparatory course, the student would be advanced to the beginning of the senior, fourth-year courses. But instead of advancing to the senior class, Lizzie opted out of the advance-standing option and enrolled in the September 1916 through February 1917 freshman-year courses.

1914/ 1915 WELTMER INSTITUTE COURSE CATALOG
The State Historical Society of Missouri (SHSMO) Artifact
(Courtesy of the Bushwhacker Museum, Nevada, Mo.)

The 1916-1917 courses would have followed the same guidelines as the prior year (above). Note the restrictions of students not allowed to work while attending school:

Students will not be able to earn their expenses while attending school. The short time required by thoroughly concentrating the attention of the class on their studies saves each student more money than he could expect to earn during a more extended course which would not require his systematic and regular attention.

Registering for the second-half year, instead of the first, required students to remain for seven months instead of six. This was due to the shutdown over Christmas, which required additional room and board for the student. Lizzie more than likely welcomed the break as it allowed time to study. Due to the fact that she received her first-year diploma in November 1916, it is believed that she signed up for the clinical portion of the fourth-year "advanced-standing" option and earned extra credits during the holiday break.

The clinical portion for each senior student, including the advanced-standing pupils, required that they accept twenty different cases, plus provide a written case history, diagnosis, and a report of all treatments given. In addition to this requisite, the student had to give a total of two-hundred treatments. Their records had to reflect full attendance in all their courses, a final exam, and a thesis of no less than 8,000 words on the theory and practice of Suggestive Therapeutics.[4] With Lizzie's experience and osteopathic skills, plus magnetic healing knowledge learned from her father, she would have been an asset to the institute when treating paying patients in the clinic.

THE FOUR YEARS comprised of specific courses for the freshman, sophomore, junior, and senior years. For students to move from first year to second, they had to receive satisfactory grades in the majority of the courses and complete the required total hours for that year. From second to third year, and third to fourth, they also had to pass a yearly exam.

Examinations in all subjects and for all course years were at the end of each term. Anyone who failed, could retake the examination at no charge within a six-month period. Before receiving a diploma for that year, the following had to be achieved: completion of both semester courses, acceptable classroom attendance, and passing grades in all of the course exams.

Seventeenth Annual Catalogue of the
Weltmer School and Sanitarium

and

Ninth Annual Announcement of the
Weltmer Institute
of
Suggestive Therapeutics

1914-1915

Nevada, Missouri, U. S. A.

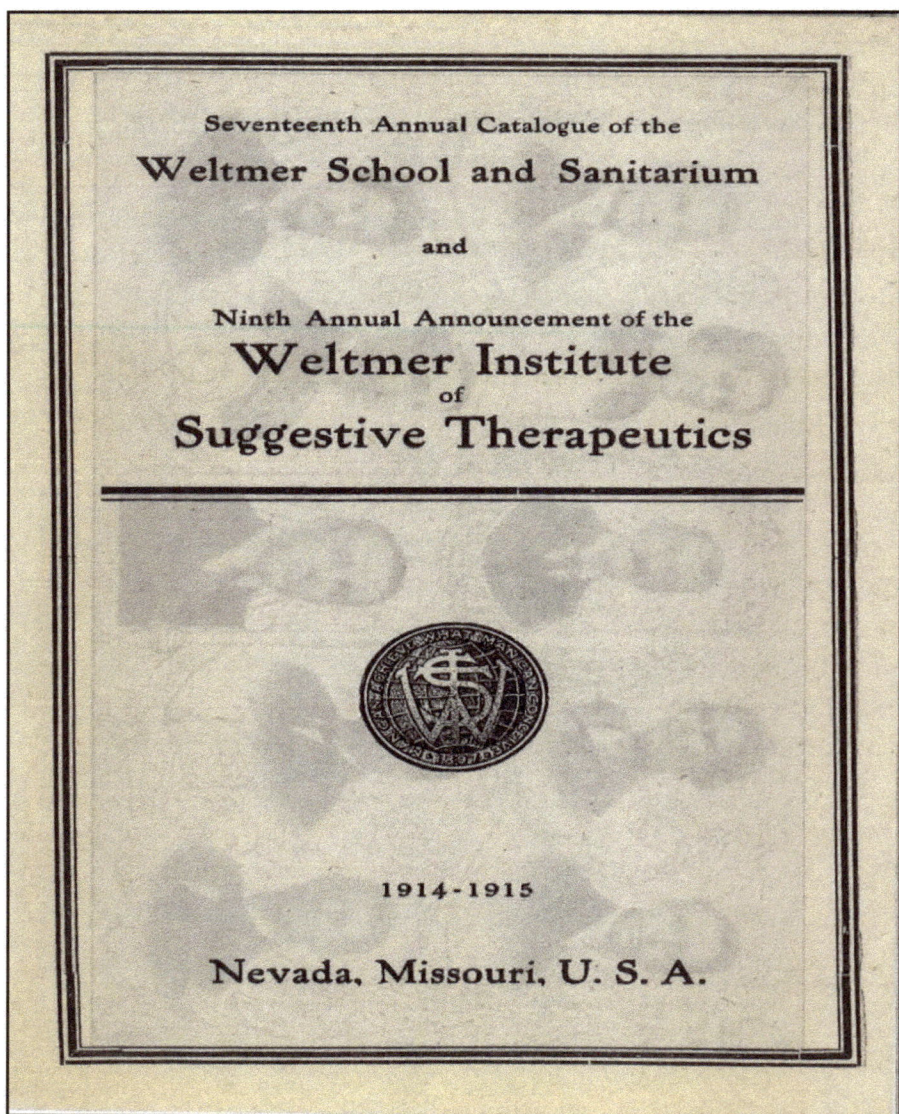

1914/ 1915 WELTMER INSTITUTE COURSE CATALOG
The State Historical Society of Missouri (SHSMO) Artifact
(Courtesy of the Bushwhacker Museum, Nevada, Mo.)

9
WELTMER INSTITUTE

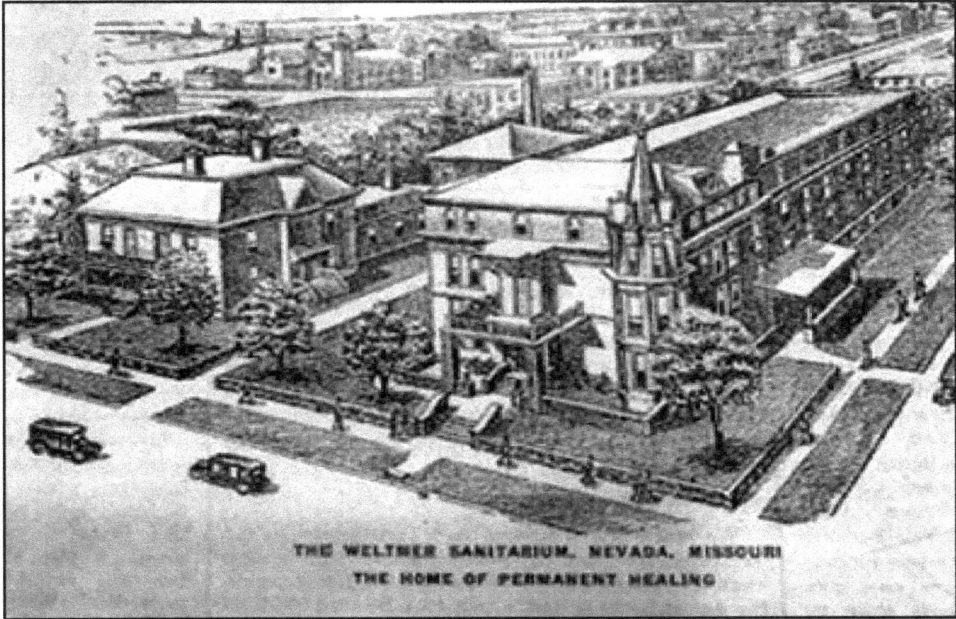

THE WELTMER SANITARIUM, NEVADA, MISSOURI
THE HOME OF PERMANENT HEALING

SKETCH OF WELTMER INSTITUTE & SANITARIUM
(Courtesy of the Bushwhacker Museum, Nevada, Mo.)

THE CAMPUS, on the corner of Austin and Ash Streets, spanned for what seemed a full city block and much larger than Lizzie had anticipated. The main building's basement no longer housed Turkish baths. It now accommodated the provisions store, kitchen, and dining rooms, plus general class rooms and clinical laboratories. In addition to stairs, all floors were connected by a freight elevator and had up-to-date amenities: hot and cold water, steam heat, electric lights, telephone, and bubbling fountains on each floor.

The first floor held the reception hall, parlor, writing room, general offices, book store, reference library, and staff offices. The second floor provided modern rooms for guests, patients, and hospital cases. The third-floor lecture hall was used daily by each-year class as depicted in the January 13, 1900 "Open House at Weltmer Institute," *Nevada Daily Mail:*

The third story occupying the entire length of the building is the spacious and elegant lecture room. This is the largest and most convenient auditorium in the city. The auditorium will be exclusively for lectures. Handsome opera chairs have been placed in this department for the convenience of the students.

There was also a two-story annex with private rooms for patients and students and a basement, which was used as the laboratory for the advanced classes.

MONDAY, SEPTEMBER 4, 1916 was the first day that Lizzie officially started courses at the institute. Some of the students reported to the lecture hall for an introductory and instructions to purchase textbooks and supplies. By midmorning, they may have headed to their classes to meet their instructors. For some courses, lessons would have started a day or two later. This is based on an excerpt of a previous-year letter from S.A. Weltmer: "The regular date of enrollment is September 1st, and the body of the class is now enrolled and will organize and settle down to regular lessons about the 6th."[1]

Lizzie's first-year courses were divided into two three-month semesters of 360 hours each:

- Psychology (general), 60 hours. Lectures and quizzes from Weltmer text.
- Anatomy, 60 hours. Lectures and quizzes, including demonstrations in Osteology from text by Cunningham.
- Physics, 60 hours. Lectures, quizzes, and laboratory work from Daniell text.
- Biology and Evolution, 60 hours. Lectures, quizzes, and laboratory from texts by Weltmer and McFarland.
- Embryology, 60 hours. Lectures and quizzes from text by McMurrich, micro-scopic study from embryological specimens and slides.
- Self-Interpretation, 60 hours. Lectures on the Greek dictum— "Know thyself."

These classes were nothing like what Lizzie's father had taken to earn his diploma. With these new teachings, the institute was modeled after a medical school. All freshman, sophomore, and junior classes had to earn 120 hours of anatomy each year to advance to the next, which included dissections of the human body.

The Missouri State Anatomical Board disposed of all unclaimed bodies from the state institutions and other sources. All recognized schools of the State received material based on a percentage of enrollment. A member of the faculty had to be a Secretary of the Board as well as the school to receive the required material for the anatomy classes.[2]

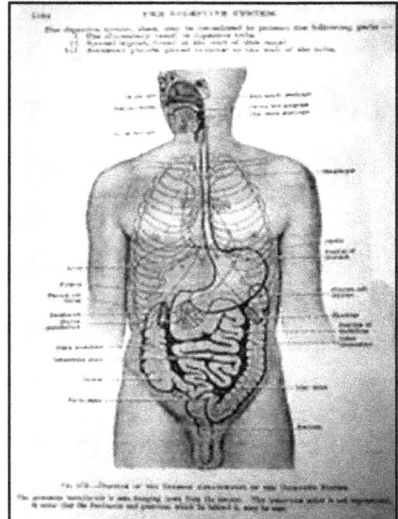

Cunningham Text Book Digestive System Diagram
(Courtesy of National Archive Digital Collection, public domain)

THE ANATOMY course was taught in three specific subjects: splanchnology, dissection, and regional anatomy.

Spanchnology, the study of the visceral organs, such as: digestive, urinary, respiratory, was taught from the Cunningham text with charts and models with demonstrations on cadavers. The abdominal and thoracic viscera were removed from the bodies and studied through a microscope. As part of this study, students had to make drawings and document their findings. Ear, nose, and throat were studied in a similar manner. The purpose: to acquaint the student with the organ's structure and better determine a patient's ailment and treatment.

Dissection was the chief teaching method to study the anatomy, biology, histology, and embryology. All instruments and material used in regular work were provided at no extra charge to the student, including the reference library and laboratories. However, any special dissection work was an extra expense. [3]

MEDICAL COLLEGES VIEWED dissection necessary for scientific advancement and inquiry. The same appeared true for the Weltmer Institute. Before the discovery of formaldehyde's tissue preservation in the 1890's, various methods to prolong putrefaction of the body were used: whiskey, brandy, and even metals like mercury or zinc.[4]

Techniques developed in the Victorian era produced treelike branches of the lungs, blood vessels, and lymphatic system after injection with colored resin or wax. Bones were bleached in the sun or dyed to highlight their shapes and shadows, and organs were preserved in jars filled with wine and turpentine.[5] Specimens of this type were also used in the Weltmer teachings.

Lizzie's records revealed that she completed 80 hours of human body dissection. Her initial reaction to handling a cadaver is unknown, but she persevered and completed the course. Students were prepped on expected anxieties, but how to overcome the emotion would be based on the individual. Lizzie's age and life experiences, plus her calm, stoic personality may have given her an edge over a younger student. One would guess that she viewed dissection as a scientific endeavor and may have prayed for the once-living cadaver, thanking him or her for their contribution to helping others.

Elizabeth Blackwell, the first American Physician to earn a medical degree on January 23, 1849, provided a colorful description her first dissection of a human wrist: "The beauty of the tendons and exquisite arrangement of this part of the body struck my artistic sense. I begin to think there is more love of science in me than I have hitherto suspected." [6]

It is believed that Lizzie had similar views. She was detailed in her thoughts and meticulous in all that she did as was documented by John Snyder in his 1894 letter. It is known that Lizzie had a quest to learn and performing dissections would have allowed her a close-up study of the human body from a scientific perspective.

WELTMER ADVERTISED THAT the school had the most modern microscopes, microtomes, Xray machines, slide films, and all apparatus necessary for preparing the tissue. All laboratory work was done under direct supervision of trained specialists. Osteology, equally important, was taught from skeletons, disarticulated bones, charts, drawings, models, and prepared specimens. The skull and spinal column in relation to the brain and the spinal cord was studied closely. Myology, Neurology, and Arthrology were taught through demonstrations and prepared specimens of ligaments and cartilages. Neurology, which was the anatomy of the nervous system, held a special interest to Lizzie. Based on her notes, she treated many with this condition. Weltmer instructors believed there was a vital connection between the function of the brain and all other organs. Nerve tracings were covered in the dissection and assisted by faculty for what was referred to as delicate work. It is known that medical doctors attended the university and presumed that some also taught these courses.

PHYCHOLOGY was covered in all of the year classes. The lab was fitted with items for proper experimentations: kymograph, ergograph, color mixers, test cards, puzzle pictures, plus other devices. It was divided into three class types:

- General psychology, which was the study of the mental process.
- Experimental psychology, most of the study was done in the laboratory.
- Applied psychology with the practice of Suggestive Therapeutics. The basic principle was that the mind controlled the functions of the body.

PHYSIOLOGY was only offered to the freshmen, sophomore, and junior classes, and taught in increments from the Dearborn text. In preparation for this course, the student was required to complete 60 hours in Biology. By having knowledge of the physiologic processes and anatomic relations in animal and plant life, the student was provided a better understanding of the human organism. The course covered physiology of circulation, lymph, respiration, digestion and metabolism, muscle, and of the cerebro-spinal and sympathetic nervous system.

Weltmer believed that the sympathetic system was more responsive to mental activity than any other physical structure. Emotions, such as anger, despair, fear, and jealousy had a negative effect on the system, but hope, joy, and love stimulated it. He also thought that both types of emotions influenced the blood's circulation. Weltmer had the distinction of being the first to teach the physiological fact that many of the diseases of humanity could be directly traced to these emotions. He stated that it was notable that the most advanced systems of medicine were based upon the therapeutic value of the blood, citing serum-therapy and opo-therapy as examples.[7]

PHYSICS, 120 hours for the freshman class only, provided a full understanding of physical laws in relationship of man to his environment. It was accomplished through lectures, quizzes, and laboratory work. In conjunction to the physics course, chemistry was taught the next year. Both aligned to the requirements of the State Examining Boards.

EMBRYOLOGY, another freshman-only class, was taught the first semester of the first year through lectures, quizzes, and laboratory study of embryonic specimens and slides.

BIOLOGY AND EVOLUTION were taught together throughout the year to provide the student an understanding of the origin of the inherent vital, physical, and mental forces in all living organisms.

SELF-INTERPRETATION consisted of lectures by Professor Weltmer to his students and sanitarium patients. He would speak openly about the inner-nature of man; of his powers, his possibilities, and his relations to his Source. His mission was to teach the student to know their own nature and redirect latent powers of their deeper self. His message was to trust their intelligent faith in themselves, in Nature, and in Nature's God.

Self-culture was included in this course and taught my Professor Weltmer's son, Ernest Weltmer. The lectures and exercises included: relaxation, physical culture, personal hygiene, social usages, mental culture, correct speech, and ethical and moral culture. The objective was to provide a comprehensive plan for the student to fit into any society and make the best use of their faculties.

NOVEMBER 25, 1916, LIZZIE received her diploma as a Suggestotherapist, showing completion of the first-year courses. She remained in Nevada over the Thanksgiving and Christmas breaks and spent most of her time in the research library or working extra hours in the clinics, which counted as credit and may have been why she received her diploma early.

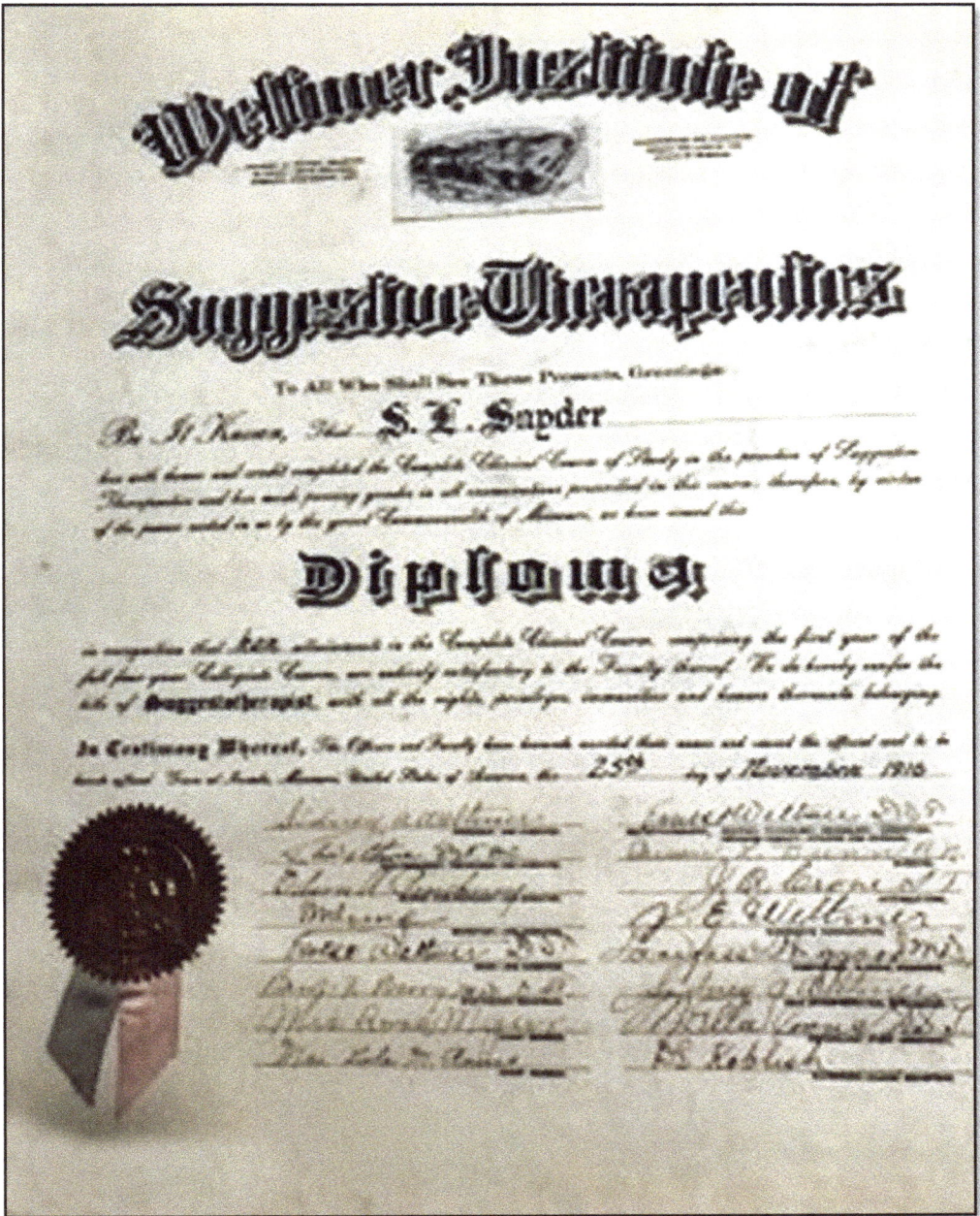

WELTMER INSTITUTE OF SUGGESTIVE THERAPEUTICS DIPLOMA
Lizzie's First-year Diploma
November 25, 1916
Signed by Sidney and Ernest Weltmer, plus others
(Author's collection)

February 22, 1917, Lizzie completed 299 hours of her second-semester requirements, including 31 additional hours of dissection. Her grade average was 90.

With the completion of this first-year course, she headed home after being gone for almost eight months.

Weltmer Institute of Suggestive Therapeutics
Second-Semester Completed Hours
(Author's collection)

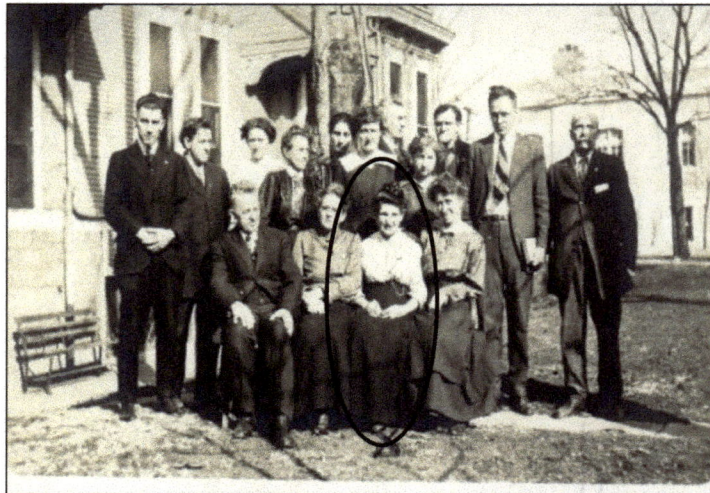

Weltmer Classmates
(Lizzie front row, 3rd from left)
(Author's collection)

WITH SUGGESTIVE THERAPEUTICS and Applied Psychology, Weltmer's fundamental belief was that if an individual was properly informed, they would think the thought that caused the healing, no matter what the affliction might be. He further stated, "We treat the mental state. We do not treat the symptoms; we direct our efforts toward the removal of the cause.[8] Excerpt from Article One: "Duties of the Suggestive Therapeutist to their patients:" [9]

- Therapeutist should always be mindful of the high character of their mission and of the responsibilities which they incur by entering the profession.

- Must never lose sight that the patient committed to his care is not normal and that seldom the friends and relatives are entirely so because of the anxiety incident on sickness.

- The obligation of secrecy.

- Frequent visits are sometimes required and it is necessary for regularity. Always be punctual.

- Suggestive Therapeutics is based on hope and must avoid gloomy prognostications. If necessary, the healer must give notice to dangerous manifestations to relatives, guardians or friends or the patient himself.

- Therapeutist should remember that they are ministers of hope and comfort to the sick.

- No patient should be abandoned because the disease or malady is of the so-called incurable nature.

- Therapeutist should be a counsellor of, as well as a minister to, the sick and suffering, plus promote and strengthened a good resolution of those suffering with consequences of evil conduct.

**WELTMER INSTITUTE
SUGGESTIVE THERAPEUTICAL ASS'N**
(Author's collection)

10
LIZZIE'S RETURN

RETURNING HOME to Hoquiam in March 1917, Lizzie barely had time to regroup before the United States had entered into World War 1 on April 6, 1917. War alone was worrisome, but more so to Lizzie and other local parents, whose sons had joined the Navy Reserve in 1914. Rumors spread that they'd soon be shipped overseas. Lizzie tried to keep positive and prayed that Lester and his friends wouldn't be called to the fight. Her hopes quickly faded with his last visit off base January 1918, informing her he'd be shipping out in early spring.

THE WAR, often referred to as the First World War or the Great War, officially started in 1914, five months after a Bosnian-Serb student assassinated the Austro-Hungarian heir, Archduke Franz Ferdinand and his wife. Austria-Hungary blamed Serbia. Diplomacy was tried, but failed, and on July 28, 1914 Austria-Hungary declared war. Russia came to Serbia's defense, and by August 4th, both blocs drew in their alliances.

The first alliance was the "Triple Entente" made up by Great Britain, France, and Imperial Russia. The second bloc was called the "Triple Alliance" of Germany, Austria-Hungary, and Italy, but later changed to the "Central Powers" when the Young Turks of the Ottoman Empire joined after they had carried out a surprise attack on Russia's Black Sea. Following this attack, Russia, France, and Britain declared war on the Ottomans. In April 1915, Italy switched sides and joined Britain, France, Russia, and Serbia, forming the "Allies of World War 1." It wasn't until Germany's unrestricted submarine warfare on the Allied Navy that the United States was pulled into the war on April 6, 1917.

By the end of the war, nine million had been killed in battle plus over five-million civilians. Also rearing its head was the 1918 Spanish-flu pandemic. Little did Lizzie know that this pandemic would impact her abroad as well as at home.

LIZZIE REOPENED HER healing practice in phases. First, concentrating on her long-standing patients and introducing new treatments learned at the Weltmer Institute. It was during this period that she began researching electrotherapy.

Electrotherapy was not taught at the Weltmer Institute, but dated back to the 1700's. Electrical energy for medical needs was first generated through the use of Leyden jars. Later, friction machines, and then, battery-operated devices. By mid-century, it was a viable treatment for tuberculosis, epilepsy, and other diseases. Since Lizzie had never mastered hypnosis, she hoped electrotherapy would aid with relaxation as well as physical therapy and was advertised to manage chronic pain and increase blood circulation too.

It is unknown how much she paid for the Bionopath machine, but it was valued as one of the key components of her practice and saved among her belongings. With the addition of this machine plus other medical devices, such as a blood-pressure cuff and a stethoscope and her expanded skills, she transformed her healing practice into a drugless clinic, offering a wide array of treatments from a simple sore throat to the more complicated Weltmer "Laying on of Hands." She even performed chiropractic services learned from her mechano-therapy degree and from helping her father in his healing practice.

The Bionopath machine was described as bionic ionization—the science of life and perpetual youth. The pamphlet stated that bionic ionization was not a germicide. It further declared that the rays produced by the machine harmonized with the body's own ionization intensity and was a recharge of the run-down human battery.

The average treatment ranged from twenty to thirty minutes, and according to the pamphlet, impossible to overtreat as bionic ionization was purely constructive and harmless. Daily treatments were advised.

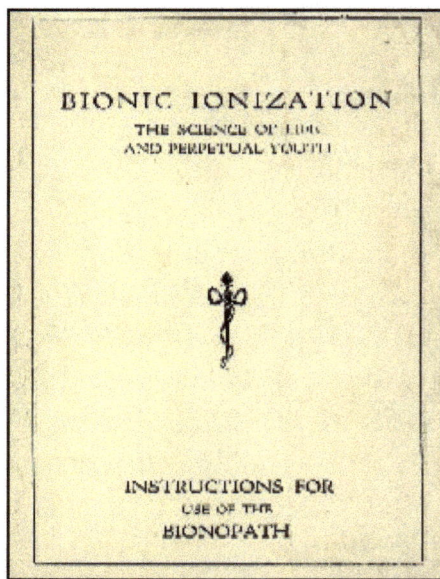

BIONIC IONIZATION
THE SCIENCE OF LIFE
AND PERPETUAL YOUTH

INSTRUCTIONS FOR
USE OF THE
BIONOPATH

(Author's collection)

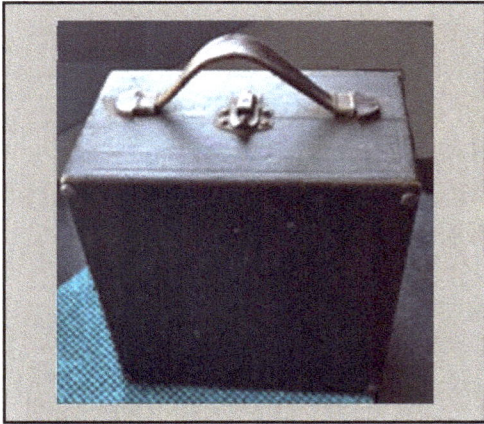

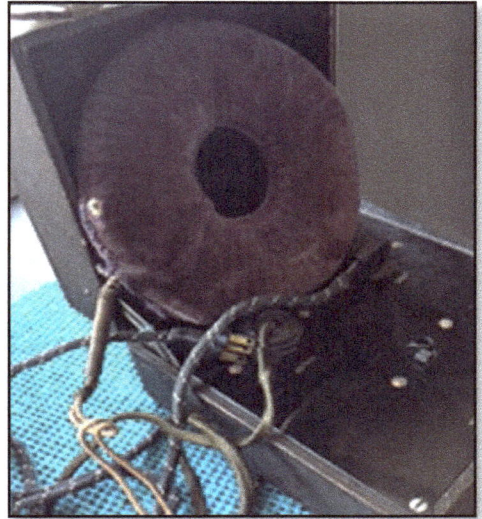

Bionopath Machine
(Author's collection)

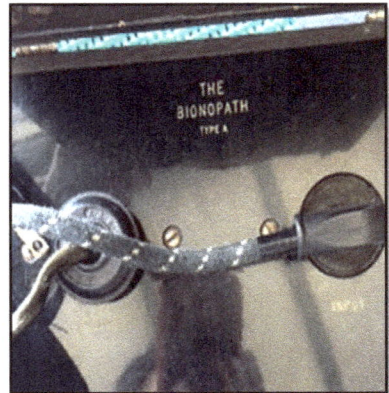

Bionopath instructions for connecting:

- The wire attached to the round applicator must be plugged into the socket of the instrument marked output.
- The other wire marked input is plugged into any electric light socket supplying 110 volts.
- By turning the switch to "on" the instrument is in operation.
- A very slight vibration will be felt in the round applicator.

Giving treatments:

- Best taken while reclining on a cot or bed.
- Place the applicator under the user next to the spine. (Not necessary to be next to the skin, as the rays penetrate the clothing, but all metals such as corsets or watches should be removed.)
- For conditions in the region of the stomach, lungs, liver, head, and kidneys or merely lowered vitality, place the application to the spine at the base of the neck.
- Intestines, pelvic region or lower extremities, place the application to the lower portion of the spine.

101

- However, the application can be placed to any part of the body with wonderful results.

It is unknown how her patients responded to the treatment. One could guess that some might have been fearful of electricity buzzing through their bodies. At any rate, it was an option for those who were brave enough to try.

WHEN LESTER shipped out in February 1918 for WW1, he was stationed in San Francisco before sailing overseas. His final destination was at the U.S. Naval Air Station, La Trinité, France.

One can only imagine Lizzie's mixed emotions: love, worry, and excitement, plus tears when she received her first overseas letter. Even more so when she saw that it was a Mother's Day card of a mother with her soldier son.

The card contained six pages of poems. *Mother O'Mine* by Rudyard Kipling was included.

Lester's message:

Dear Mother –

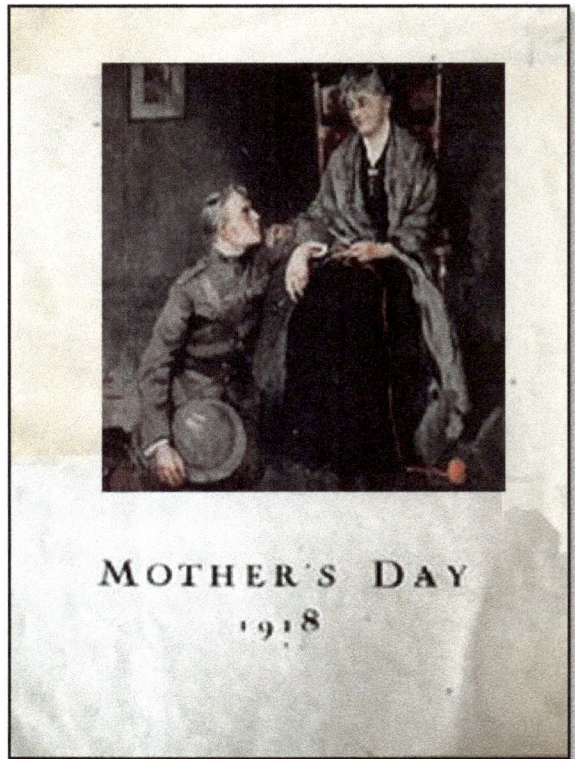

(Author's collection)

> *Tho this was late in getting started to you because I just obtained it today. It contains so many of my thoughts that I am going to let it be my letter to you today and this be only a little side issue.*
>
> *Mother O'Mine is my favorite expression and seeing that the author is somewhat older than I, I guess I stole it from him, instead of he from me.*

Received a nice letter from Will and Myrtle today. Mother dear, hope you will be pleased to note that my rate now is one notch higher than it was, now being Seaman 1st class. We received a big mail today, but I did not get one from Etta, but will probably in the next mail, I hope so at least. Remember me to Mrs. Patred and Emma Larson. Love to all and bushels for your own dear self. [1]

Son, Les
Les. H. Hanson (Sea)
U.S. Naval Air Station, La Trinite
c/o Postmaster, New York

Lizzie had a special bond with William Jr. and Lester from their hard times at the boardinghouse. As much as her boys relied on her for strength and guidance, they were her anchor too. Family letters and pictures reveal the closeness that remained between the three throughout their lives.

Lizzie's reply, May 1918:

My dear boy:
Your father says to tell you that he will give his son to his country, but that he will be (never missed whist!) if he will give all his new suspenders. He says you pinched three pair from the top drawer of his bureau—he adds that he "is onto your curves." Nora says you were very wise to take them and she would give you all of hers, if she had any!

Betty says to tell you that she hears Jack Ellis sails next week—I know just how his mother will feel for those ten days while he is crossing. But she wouldn't have had him stay at home, any more than I would have had you! All the same, she won't have a good night's sleep until she hears he has landed...I keep thinking what a different world it will be to mothers, when you all come marching home again!

And when you do come marching home old fellow bring me back the same boy I gave my country, true & clean & gentle & brave. You must do this for your father & me & Betty & Nora—& most of all, for the daughter you will give to me one of these days!

Dear, I don't know whether you have even met her yet—but never mind that! Live for her or if God wills, die for her—but do either with courage — "with honor & clean mirth!" But I know you will come back to me— [2]

Mother—

Betty, Nora, Emma, and Jack were Lester's childhood friends. Lester considered John Snyder his father. The daughter you will give to me was a euphemism for Lester's future wife. Lizzie must have suspected that girl might be Etta, who lived in Seattle and was mentioned in Lester's letter. What Lizzie didn't know, but later revealed, Lester and Etta had married on January 10, 1918, several weeks before he shipped out. Will and Myrtle were Lester's brother, William Jr. and his wife. Mrs. Patred, a close family friend and often referred to as Auntie, was married to F.A. Patred, president of the Hoquiam Steam Boiler Works, who was also a fraternal member of the Masons with John Snyder. Mrs. Patred was a healer in her own right, which cemented her friendship to Lizzie even more.

Mrs. Patred and Lizzie with Lester several weeks before he shipped out for WWI

(January 1918)
(Author's collection)

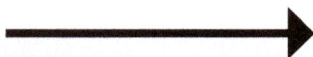

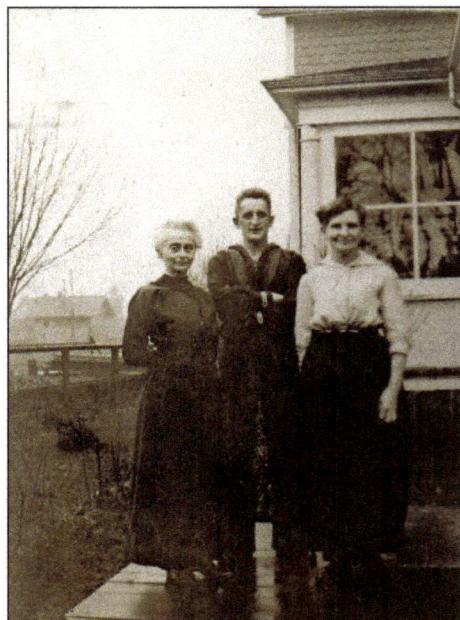

WHEN NEWS THAT the 1918 Spanish-flu pandemic was spreading throughout Europe and infecting our troops, Lizzie's worry for Lester intensified. It had hit home in August when a trainload of Navy seamen from Philadelphia arrived to Washington State with symptoms of chills, fever, and fatigue. Most of the men recovered quickly, but by late September, another military base, Camp Lewis, 45 miles south of Seattle, reported men developing pneumonia.

First of October, a large number of cases were reported at the naval training base at the University of Washington, where Lester had been stationed. One cadet died and 700 others were ill with more than half in the hospital.

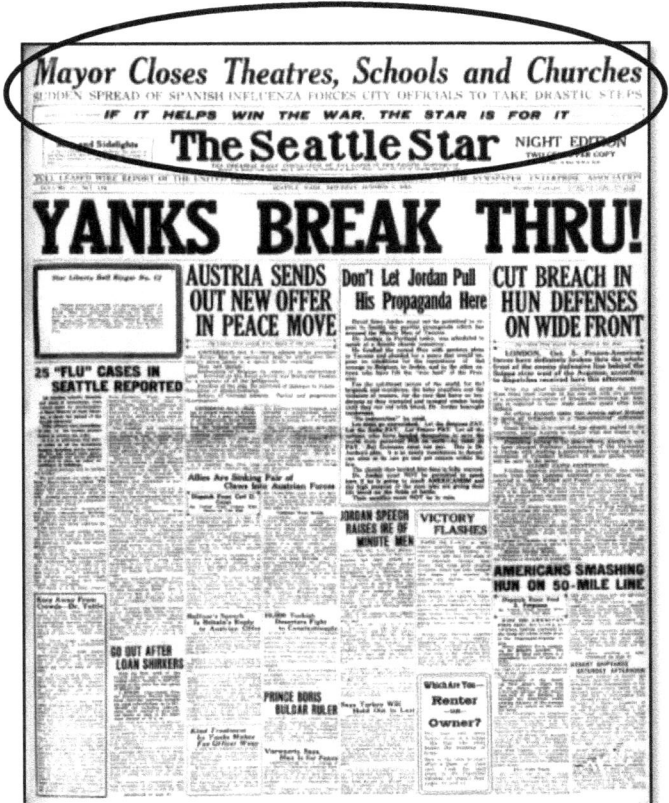

THE SEATTLE STAR
(Courtesy Library of Congress Digital Collection, Newspapers, public domain)
October 8, 1918

October 6, 1918, Seattle churches were halted and theaters, poolrooms, libraries, cafes and restaurants were prohibited. Public schools closed. By the end of the month, masks were mandated for anyone shopping at a store, boarding a streetcar or in any other public situation coming in contact with another person. [3]

The largest cities were impacted the most, but the virus trickled down to smaller communities too. The first news of the virus hitting Grays Harbor, where Lizzie lived, was in early October with the death of a 28-year-old pharmacist from pneumonia in his Aberdeen home. Shortly after, women were encouraged to enroll as nurses or as volunteers to help those with virus-stricken households. [4]

It is known that Lizzie and her daughter, Florence, had volunteered at the local Red Cross. After graduation, Florence enrolled in the U.S. Student Nurse Reserve and worked as a volunteer at the hospital. She later became a nurse.

U. S. STUDENT NURSE RESERVE
COUNCIL OF NATIONAL DEFENSE
WASHINGTON, D. C.

A. CERTIFICATE OF HIGH SCHOOL STUDY.
(To be filled out and signed by the principal or some other authorized officer of the High School.)

This is to certify that the applicant, Miss *Florence Snyder*

(1) Was a student in *Hoquiam High School* at *Hoquiam, Wash.*
(Name of secondary school.) (Location.)

for a period of *four* years, beginning *Sept. 1st*, 19*14*, and

ending *June 7*, 19*18*

(2) Was duly graduated in *June*, 19*18*

(3) Or completed satisfactorily the subjects indicated below.

(4) Left the institution in good standing.

(5) Do you recommend her admission to a school of nursing?

	SUBJECTS.	WEEKS A YEAR.	PERIODS A WEEK.	MINUTES A PERIOD.	STANDING, PER CENT.
First Year. Completed or not completed. Date *1914 1915*	*Eng. I & II*	*38*	*5*	*45*	*77*
	Alg. I & II	*38*	*5*	*45*	*70*
	Anct. Hist.	*38*	*5*	*45*	*80*
	Type Writing	*19*	*5*	*45*	*90*
Second Year. Completed or not completed. Date *1915 1916*	*Eng. III & IV*	*38*	*5*	*45*	*70*
	Geom. I & II	*38*	*5*	*45*	*70*
	Med. Hist.	*19*	*5*	*45*	*70*
	Domestic Science	*38*	*5*	*80*	*70*
Third Year. Completed or not completed. Date *1916 1917*	*Eng. V & VI*	*38*	*5*	*45*	*75*
	Alg. Advanced	*19*	*5*	*45*	*70*
	Botany	*38*	*3*	*80*	*75*
	Physics	*38*	*5*	*80*	*70*
Fourth Year. Completed or not completed. Date *1917 1918*	*Eng. VII & VIII*	*38*	*5*	*45*	*70*
	Gen. Biology	*38*	*5*	*80*	*70*
	German 1st yr.	*38*	*5*	*45*	*70*
	U. S. Hist.	*38*	*5*	*45*	*70*
	German 2nd yr.	*38*	*5*	*45*	*75*

Date *Sept. 30*, 19*18*.

(Signed) *A. J. Bonham*

(Official title) *Principal, High School*

FLORENCE SNYDER, U.S. STUDENT NURSE RESERVE
(Author's collection)

With another uptick of cases in early December, the Red Cross was running thin and was forced to open an emergency hospital in the Eagles Hall on Seventh and J Street in Hoquiam.[5] Florence continued helping at the Red Cross. Her walk from home on First Street to the new facility was ten minutes or so. Lizzie, however, was inundated with patients of her own.

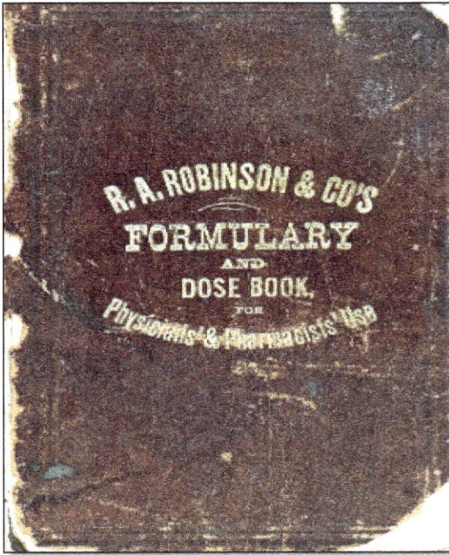

LIZZIE'S FORMULARY BOOK
(Author's collection)

When word had spread that Lizzie had completed one year of medical courses, locals began showing up on her doorstep.[6] She dusted off her formulary book from her days of working with Mr. Lee, her Chinese friend, who had created her healing garden of special herbs, beehive boxes for honey, and berries for syrups. All used for treating ailments. The book contained recipes from local plants: skunk cabbage, foxgloves, and rhubarb, ordered as fluid extracts to make syrups. Special powders, herbs, and teas would have been procured from other sources too. One page was earmarked for arrowroot recipes, which were used for inflammation and digestive disorders. This more than likely would have aided in the treatment of flu-like symptoms.

Prior to the war, Lizzie had ordered spices and herbs from overseas and did have a stockpile on hand. It is believed that the four pounds of flour she had ordered in 1908 from the Baroda Camp in India was arrowroot.

BARODA CAMP, INDIA
(INT'L MONEY ORDER)
(Author's collection)

107

Many of the herbal remedies, some listed in the formulary book, were developed by healers who were once tagged as wise women or witches. They had pain-killers, digestive aids, and anti-inflammatory agents. Ergot, listed in a formulary ad, was used by the healers for the pain of labor. Digitalis, for treating heart ailments.[7]

Lizzie's also prescribed beef tea for those having difficulty with digestion and offered "Essences of Meats: Beef, Mutton, and Chicken," as an alternative. It is believed that Mrs. Patred occasionally provided advice with the creation of medicinal recipes.

Mrs. Patred, pictured with Lizzie and Lester before he shipped overseas, was born in 1844 in Calumet County, Wisconsin. Her obituary, published in the *Escanaba Daily Press*, May 10, 1923, stated that she was well known to a great many Escanaba people. Lizzie noted that Mrs.

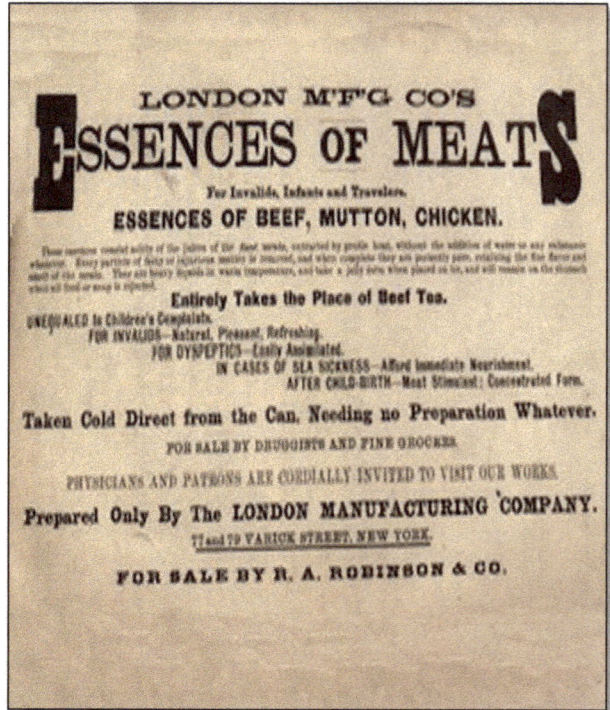

LIZZIE'S FORMULARY BOOK
(Author's collection)

Patred chronicled some of the Ojibwe treatments. The Ojibwe were one of the Anishinaabe, Algonquian-speaking tribes who had settled around the Great Lakes. They believed that everything was spiritual and viewed themselves as an element of nature and held all things of nature in high regard. Their use of plants and animals for food, clothing, and other items showed the interconnection. Those who studied to be a medicine man or medicine women used different herbs for healing as well as for enhancement of spiritual insight. Many of the ceremonial feasts included: wild rice, fresh or dried blueberries, and maple sugar.[8]

When Lester didn't tell Mrs. Patred directly that he was getting married, she was deeply hurt. Lizzie intervened and smoothed it out, but Lester had to apologize in person after he had returned home.

Excerpt, Lester's letter:

I am sorry if Auntie Patred felt hurt because I didn't tell her in exact words that Etta and I were going to be married...

LESTER'S LETTER
(Author's collection)

SEPTEMBER THROUGH the end of the year, the Spanish-flu virus had turned deadly with pulmonary edema and infections from bacterial pneumonia. Once a victim's lungs filled with fluid, they died within hours or days. The highest at risk were those between the ages of 20 and 40. In addition to her patients, Lizzie was worried for Lester. He had just turned 30.

September 8, 1918, Lester reassured his mother that he was healthy. He must have received a letter from her voicing concerns. Excerpts of his reply: "Everything is going fine. I am in the best of health."

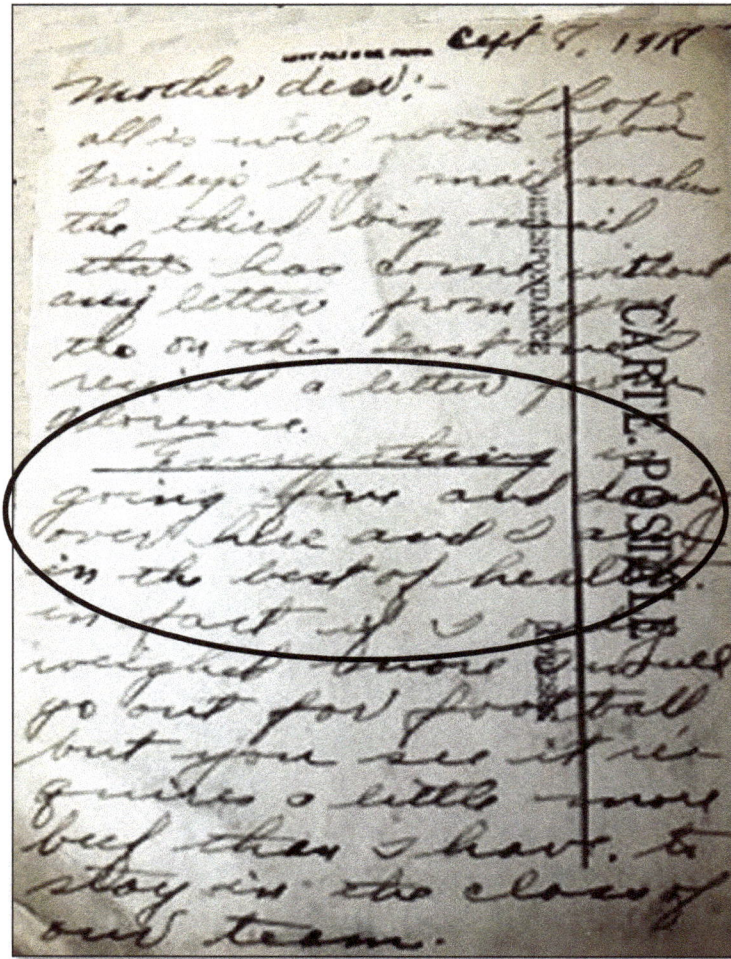

LESTER'S SEPT 8, 1918 POSTCARD
(Author's collection)

The third wave of the pandemic hit later that winter, and by spring 1919, the virus was over. The pandemic had touched nearly every community. In the end, nearly 5,000 Washingtonians had died, most between the ages of 20 and 49.[9]

11
SANIPRACTIC

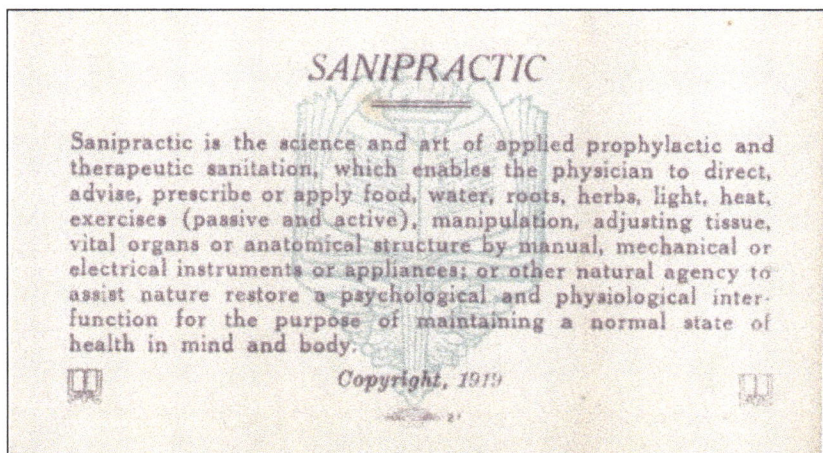

BACK OF LIZZIE'S BUSINESS CARD
(Author's collection)

Sanipractic is the science and art of applied prophylactic and therapeutic sanitation, which enables the physician to direct, advise, prescribe or apply food, water, roots, herbs, light, heat, exercises (passive and active), manipulation, adjusting tissue, vital organs or anatomical structure by manual, mechanical or electrical instruments or appliances, or other natural agency to assist nature restore a psychological and physiological inter-function for the purpose of maintaining a normal state of health in mind and body.

BY EARLY 1919, Lizzie's concerns had been eased: World War 1 had ended, the virus was in decline, and Lester's unit had sailed home, stationing him in San Francisco. During the pandemic, she had been working in more of a nursing capacity, including homeopathic treatments through the use of medicinal medicines, but followed the Weltmer teachings too. Her membership with the

Weltmer Suggestive Therapeutical Association continued, but she also sought out other methods with hopes of guiding her patients in making better choices before diseases started or progressed. When the Science of Sanipractic had been introduced by the Washington Association of Drugless Physicians, Lizzie caught a train to their headquarters in Spokane to investigate.

Sanipractic was a drugless system specific to the Pacific Northwest. It offered many of the treatments that she was already performing, including the use of natural herbs and spices but new preventive treatments too. She quickly joined their organization and enrolled in United Drugless Post Graduate fall courses taught at their Spokane institute. Prior to leaving for the courses, she received a letter, September 25, 1919, from the organization with specific instruction for spinal adjustments.

It was during this period that physicians across the states began lobbying for new laws for non-degreed healers. It is unknown if this new mandate was from the chiropractic community or the physician's lobby or caution by the United Drugless organization, itself. Nonetheless, the message was clear: she was to convey that she did not give chiropractic. Instead, was adjusting the spine in addition to other measures to give relief and to state that she was a "Sanipractic Physician." She abided by their rules, however years prior, she had studied and earned a diploma from the Mechano-Therapy College with credentials of an osteopath, which included chiropractic. In this same letter she received 100-courtesy business cards with her trade name and title, Sanipractic Physician, imprinted.

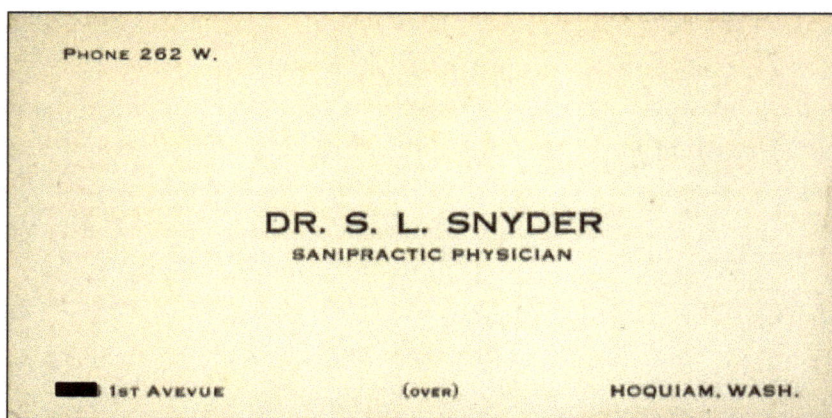

PHONE 262 W.

DR. S. L. SNYDER
SANIPRACTIC PHYSICIAN

1ST AVEVUE   (OVER)   HOQUIAM, WASH.

DR. S.L. SNYDER'S BUSINESS CARD
(Author's collection)

DR. JOHN E. LYDON, PRESIDENT   DR. S. A. AMBROSE, VICE PRESIDENT   DR. A. E. GREENE, SECRETARY   DR. T. R. THURSTON, TREASURER
SPOKANE, WASH.   TACOMA, WASH.   SEATTLE, WASH.   SPOKANE, WASH.

Washington Association of Drugless Physicians, Inc.

REPRESENTATIVES OF THE FOLLOWING SYSTEMS   HEAD OFFICE   BOARD OF DIRECTORS
310-311 AUDITORIUM BUILDING   DR. C. HALE KIMBLE, SPOKANE, WASH.
SANIPRACTIC   SPOKANE, WASH.   DR. THEO. E. OSTLUND, SEATTLE, WASH.
PHYSCULTOPATHY   SUGGESTIVE THERAPEUTICS   DR. S. SHERMAN SILVIS, SEATTLE, WASH.
MEDICAL GYMNASTICS   CHIROPRACTIC   DR. DANIEL SYMMES, SPOKANE, WASH.
AND MASSAGE   MECHANO-THERAPY   DR. F. P. LINT, CLARKSTON, WASH.
FOOD CHEMISTRY   NATUROPATHY
SWEDISH MOVEMENTS   MENTAL SCIENCE

MAKE ALL CHECKS PAYABLE TO WASHINGTON
ASSOCIATION OF DRUGLESS
PHYSICIANS, INC

Spokane, Wash., Sept. 25, 1919.

Dear Doctor:

The Washington Association of Drugless Physicians desires to inform you further relative to spinal adjustments:

Should anyone call for Chiropractic, simply state you do not give Chiropractic, but that you adjust the spine in addition to other measures to give relief to conditions which come to you for treatment; that you adjust the spine for the purpose of correcting mechanical interference with the normal function of the emunctory channels; that you align those vertebrae interfering with the lymphatic and glandular system through which the poison and effete matter drains in through and from the body, which also assists normal interfunction and sanitation of mind and body.

State to those who call that you are a Sanipractic Physician and under your name on cards or door place the term—Sanipractic (Drugless) Physician.

Enclosed one hundred cards gratis with the compliments of your Association, which should guide you in having cards printed.

Please advise how many you desire after placing your telephone number and any other subject-matter you desire on copy, sign your name and return as soon as possible and we will print same at cost. The Association is arranging to have two hundred thousand cards printed and distributed to the members who are Sanipractors and, it is needless to say, Sanipractic will be known as defined on the card, in every town in the state within a short space of time and become a household word.

We are pleased to advise that everything is going fine with the Drugless movement in the state and we have nothing to worry about.

The Association advises that every member stand back of the Washington Sanipractorium, which in reality is your institution and which will be built to provide for every practical and scientific method for the relief of human ills and betterment of public health.

In no other way can you eventually come into full recognition of your own in the drugless field, and the Drugless Practitioners generally meet the unqualified endorsement of the public, than by the construction and maintenance of such institutions. That is one of the necessary

WASHINGTON ASSOCIATION OF DRUGLESS PHYSICIANS, INC.
September 25, 1919
(Author's collection)

MANY OF THE COURSES offered by the United Drugless Post Graduate Institute, Lizzie had been practicing for years. These included: Chiropractic, Electrotherapy, Mechano-therapy, and Suggestive Therapeutics. She chose Mechano-therapy and Suggestive Therapeutics for her post-graduate studies, but her real interest was expanding her sanipractic skills, which followed in line to the naturopathic theory that most diseases were treatable or preventable through diet, exercise, and massage. Other natural approaches like hydrotherapy, a water treatment for arthritis and other related diseases, were considered naturopathic as well. She realigned her courses to include these studies.

NATUROPATHY WAS BROUGHT to America by Benedict Lust in 1896, but not without merit. Four years prior, he had arrived to New York from Germany a young man with dreams but was seized by tuberculosis. After the doctors pronounced that he'd be dead in days, he managed to return to his homeland, then on to the Bavarian village of Wörishofen, famous for its Kneippism water cures. When he regained his health, Kneipp, a priest and a healer, urged Lust to return to America to spread the Gospel of the water cure.[1]

Lust started a German periodical, then switched to English with his *Kneipp Water Cure Monthly,* but included other nature-cure therapies that he had studied during his recuperation in Germany. These included: diet, exercise, massage, sunbathing, and other drugless options. In 1901, he opened the "American School of Naturopathy" in Manhattan and offered a two-term, eighteen-month program, which would earn the graduate a degree of ND (Naturopathic Doctor).

Medical doctors blamed disease from outside elements, such as germs, but the naturopathy view was that all sickness originated within the body. This was also Weltmer's philosophy. Naturopaths also considered drugs poison, instead they used herbs.

In 1907, the official definition of naturopathy included mechanical, physical, mental, and spiritual methods. Breaking it down further, mechanical and physical vibration included: massages, manipulation, adjustment, electricity, magnetism, earth, water, air, sun, and electric light. They also endorsed hot and cold, moist and dry baths, plus fasting, dieting, physical culture, and suggestive therapeutics.[2]

Whether Lizzie realized it or not, she had already been working as a naturopath. Other courses taught at the institute were Chiropody, the treatment of feet-related ailments and Physcultopathy, a term created by bodybuilder Bernarr

Macfadden, which promoted natural foods, exercise, fasting, and even nudism, plus avoidance of all things bad: coffee, tea, alcohol and tobacco. Lizzie may have investigated these studies as well, but did not pursue.

On December 9, 1919, Lizzie earned a degree from the United Drugless Post Graduate Institute with credentials as Dr. Sarah L. Snyder, D.S.T. and M.T.D.— Suggestive Therapist and Mechano-Therapist.

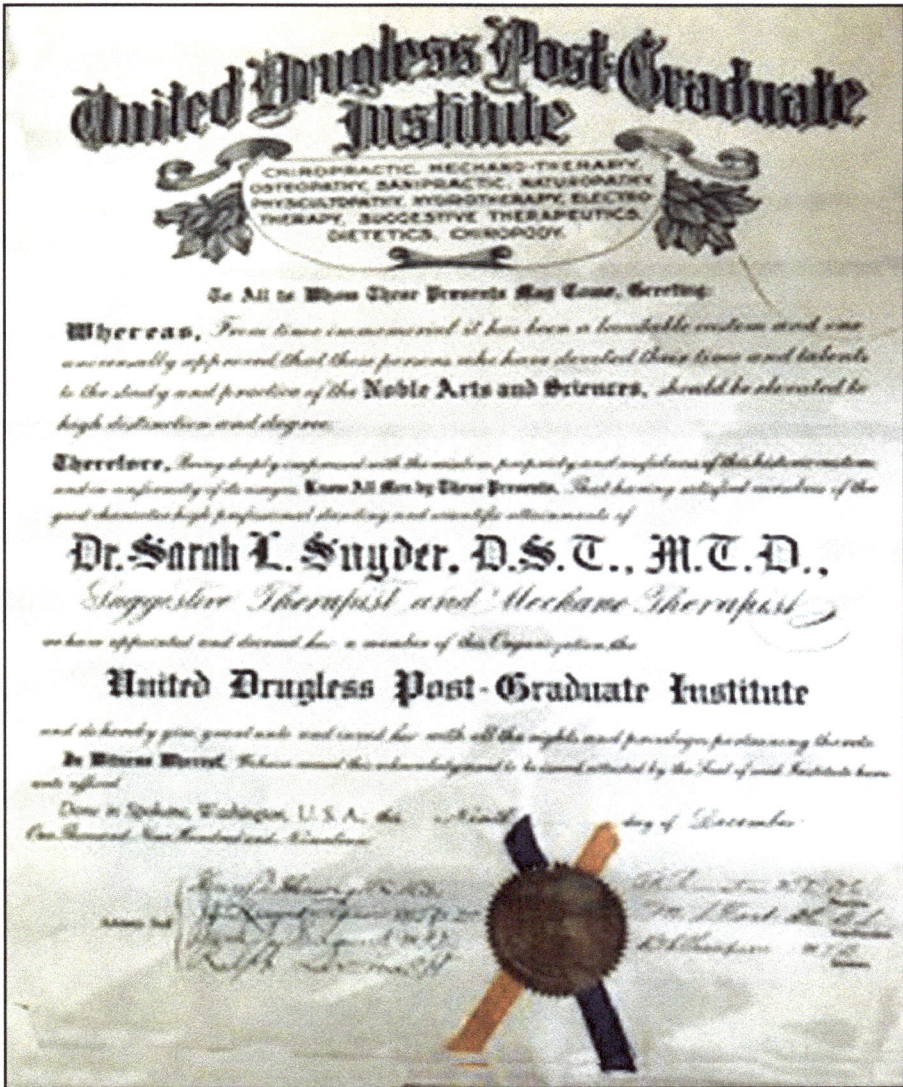

UNITED DRUGLESS POST-GRADUATE INSTITUTE
Spokane, Washington (Dec 9, 1919)
Dr. Sarah L. Snyder, D.S.T., M.T.D.
(Author's collection)

Heading home from Eastern Washington, Lizzie stopped in Seattle to visit Lester and Etta. She and Etta had been corresponding through letters, but this was their first meeting and the first time Lizzie had seen Lester since his returning home from overseas. Lizzie had planned to stay through Christmas, but remained longer after she had enrolled in the American University of Sanipractic, where she earned an honorary degree on February 12, 1920.

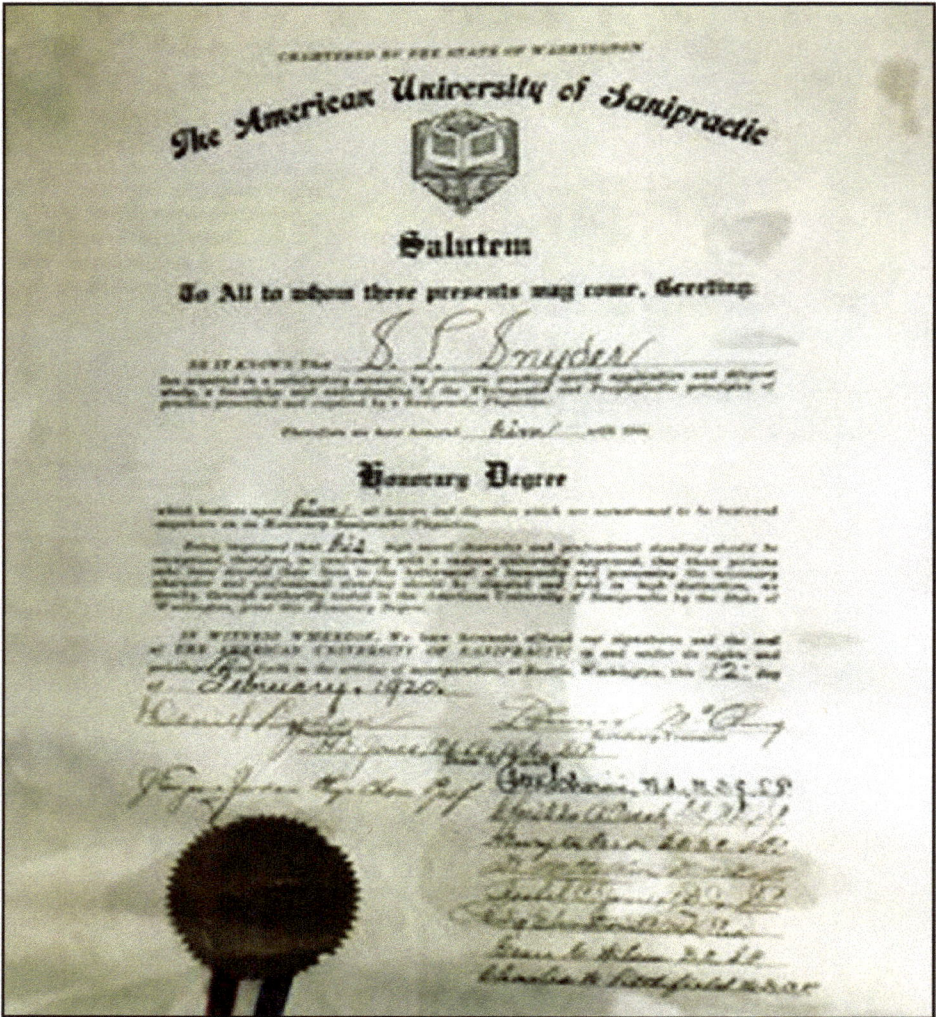

THE AMERICAN UNIVERSITY OF SANIPRACTIC
Honorary Degree
(February 12, 1920)
(Author's collection)

Prior to 1919, licensing of healers was not required, but as soon as the law was passed, Lizzie submitted the paperwork with back-up and paid the associated fees. When Washington State enacted its drugless healers' statue in 1919, the law stipulated that the Board of Drugless Examiners consist of eight practitioners: two mechano-therapists, two food scientist, two physcultopaths, and two suggestive therapists. At first, the majority of the state legislatures only granted naturopaths the right to do little more than massage.[3]

Based on Lizzie's license, it appears that the examiners had authority to issue specific licenses tied to the applicant's credentials. On February 5, 1920, Lizzie received from the State of Washington Board of Drugless Examiners a license to practice as a Suggestive Therapist with a listing of approved treatments:

Acting under authority of an Act of the Legislature, approved February 18,1919, hereby grants Sara [sic] (Sarah) L. Snyder a license to practice Suggestive Therapeutics within the following subjects: gynecology, hydrotherapy, psychology, uranalysis, dietetics, sanitation, and manual manipulations.

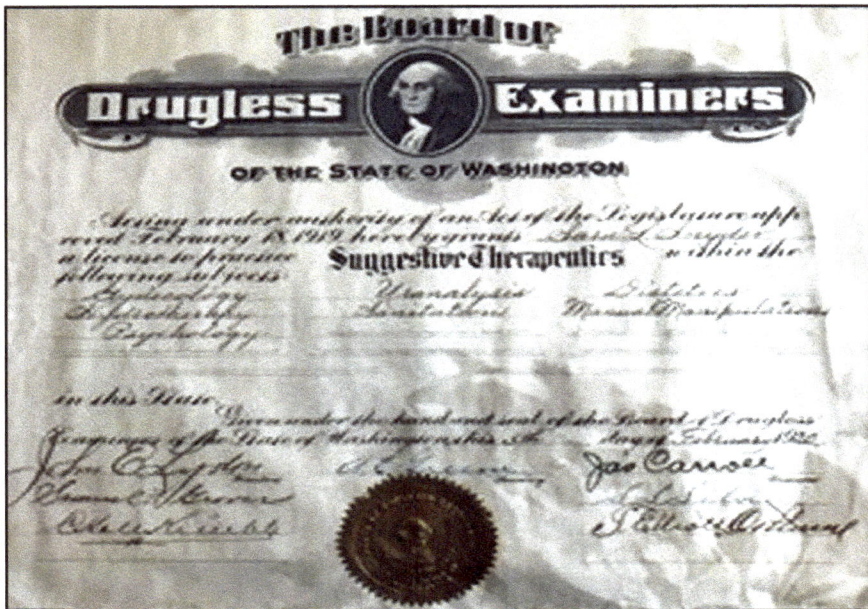

**DRUGLESS EXAMINERS
STATE CERTIFICATION
(Feb 5, 1920)**
(Author's collection)

117

On June 3, 1920, she received her membership certificate from the Washington Association of Drugless Physicians. Three weeks later, she attended their convention in Vancouver, Washington held at the Elks Temple. Not only did she meet other delegates from the Pacific coast states, she learned of new treatments and had the opportunity to view the latest in medical devices and equipment.[4]

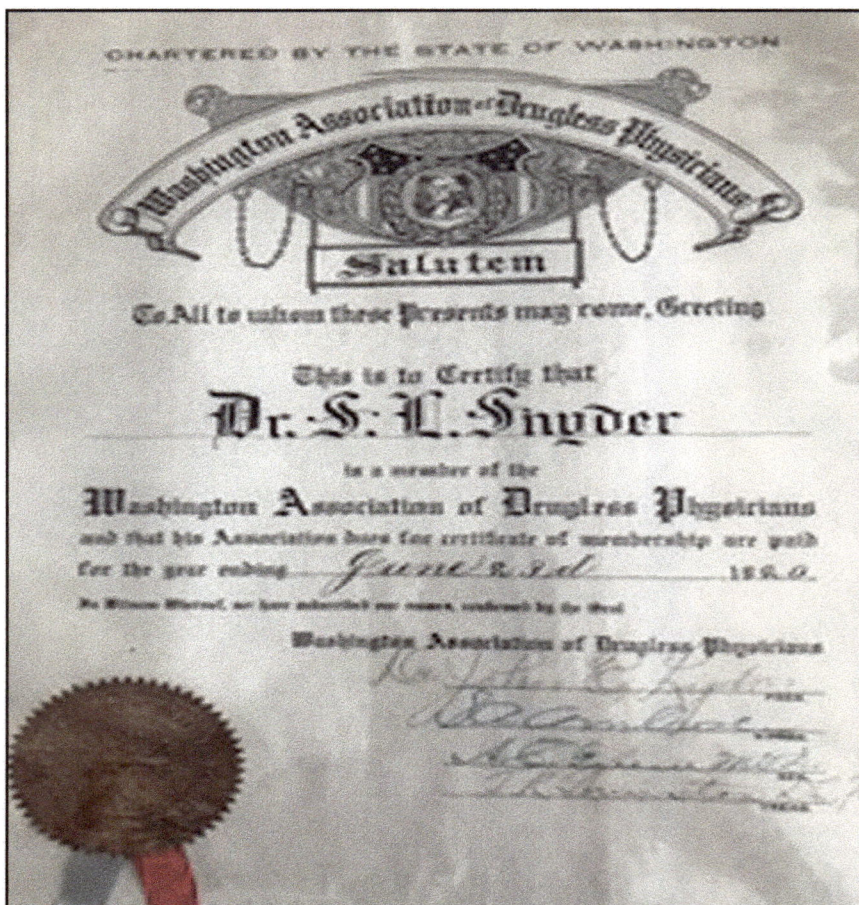

**WASHINGTON ASSOCIATION OF
DRUGLESS PHYSICIANS 1920 CERTIFICATE**
(Author's collection)

This was also the first time that Lizzie, now age 56, was listed on the 1920 census as a doctor of therapeutics.

Sarah L Snyder
in the 1920 United States Federal Census

Detail | Source

Name:	Sarah L Snyder
Age:	56
Birth Year:	abt 1864
Birthplace:	Iowa
Home in 1920:	Hoquiam Ward 3, Grays Harbor, Washington
Street:	First St.
Residence Date:	1920
Race:	White
Gender:	Female
Relation to Head of House:	Wife
Marital Status:	Married
Spouse's Name:	John B Snyder
Father's Birthplace:	Ohio
Mother's Birthplace:	Virginia
Able to Speak English:	Yes
Occupation:	Doctor
Industry:	Therapeutics
Employment Field:	Own Account
Able to read:	Yes
Able to Write:	Yes
Neighbors:	View others on page

Household Members	Age	Relationship
John B Snyder	61	Head
Sarah L Snyder	**56**	**Wife**
Lincoln L Snyder	22	Son
Florence E Snyder	21	Daughter
Ethel V Wilson	19	Niece

UNITED STATES
1920 CENSUS
(Courtesy of NARA—National Archives and Records)
(Public domain)

A letter from Seattle Supply Company, dated August, 15 1920, referencing a stethoscope that Lizzie purchased at the Vancouver convention, reassured her that the one she had procured was satisfactory, but they provided a cut (picture) of the Douglas Stethoscope if she preferred it instead. Lizzie wanting the best traded up.

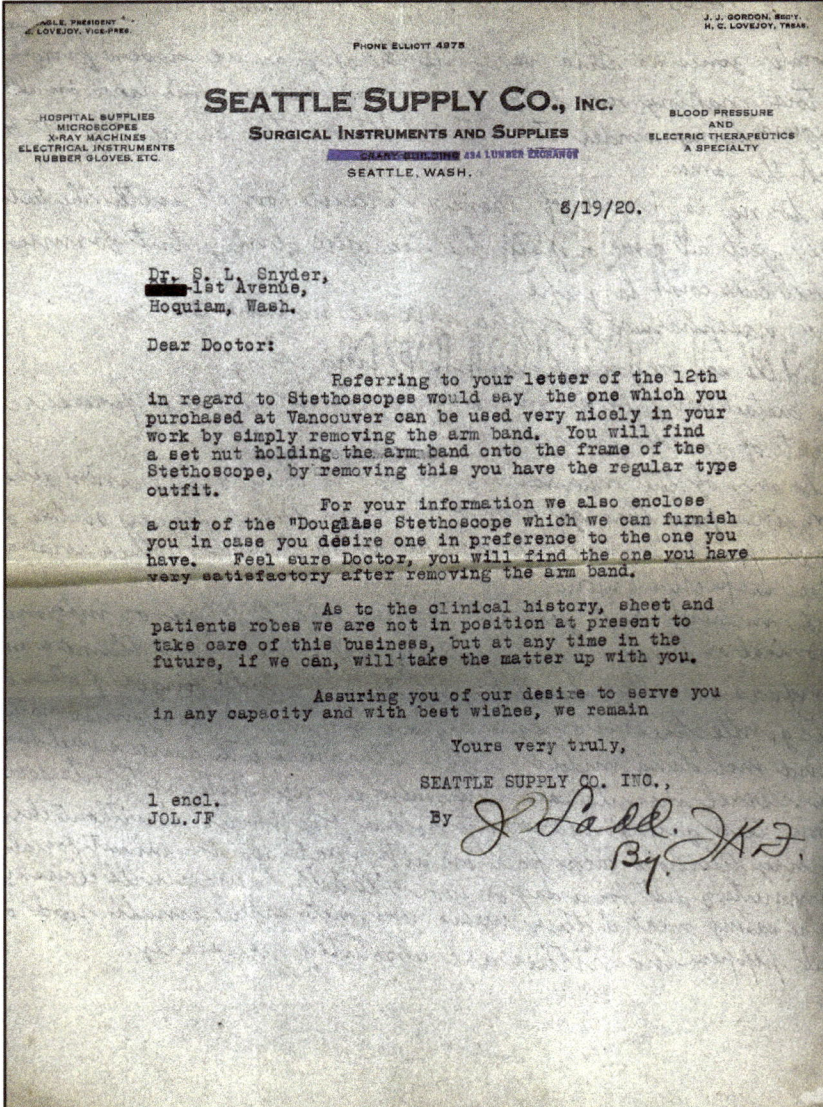

SEATTLE SUPPLY CO. INC., SEATTLE, WA
Stethoscope purchase at convention
Aug 15, 1920
(Author's collection)

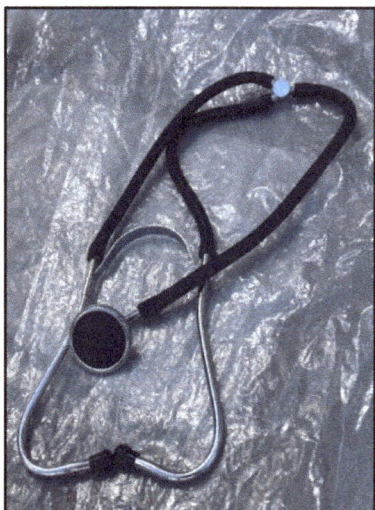

**S.L. Snyder's
Stethoscope**
(Author's collection)

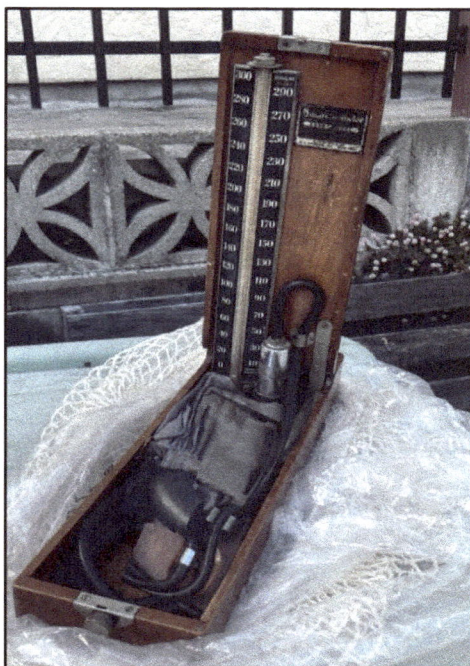

**S.L. Snyder's Baumanometer
Blood Pressure Monitor**
(S/N 93288)
(Author's collection)

Mercury sphygmomanometers, the "gold standard" because of their accuracy, was also known as the Baumanometer.

Invented by William A. Baum and first marketed in 1917, was a "must have" for Lizzie's practice.

While watching the mercury in the column and releasing the air pressure with the control valve, the practitioner would monitor the blood pressure. He'd also listen through the stethoscope.

Note: a heavy glass bulb held the mercury.

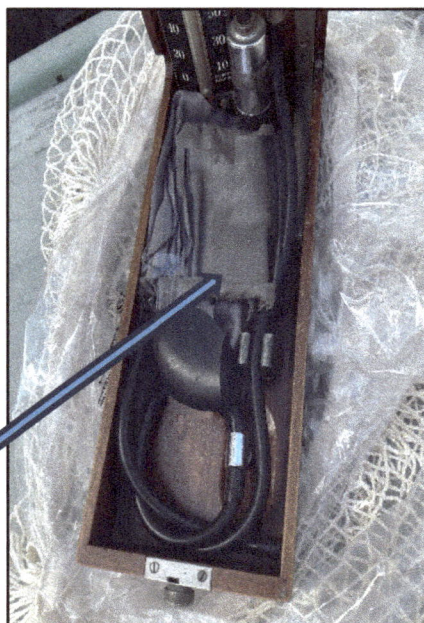

Lizzie followed Weltmer's record-keeping format as outlined in the *How to Succeed* book. One of the first requirements was the completion of the four-page diagnostic sheet. Accentuating the importance of this step, Weltmer stated:

In making the examination you must first learn enough to satisfy yourself that you understand the case and can accomplish a cure; and second, you must convince him that you do understand and that you can accomplish a cure.

WELTMER DIAGNOSTIC FORM (PAGE 1 OF 4)
National Archives (The Weltmer Institute, 1919, *How to Succeed*)
(Public domain)

Do not permit yourself to skim over any one case. If you haven't time to examine a case carefully and make a careful record of it, you haven't time to do it at all and should set another time when you will have time. [5]

Weltmer recommended other avenues to a patient if he deemed it necessary, such as surgery or chiropractic. This diagnosis sheet would have also been used for Absent Treatments: first mailed to the patient, returned to the healer, then sent back to the patient with instruction or a request for more information. Once the healer was satisfied with the results, he'd schedule a date and time for them to synchronize minds.

The questionnaire probed into such items as medicines, vices—tobacco or drinking—ailments, fatigue, exercise, eating habits, and water consumption. Plus, a remarks section for the patient to expand explanation of items listed or something not covered. It was advised that the healer make the examination without advancing any theories beforehand and say as little as possible. In doing so, Weltmer believed that the patient would be put into a receptive mindset to take treatments after witnessing the thoroughness of the examination.

Weltmer stressed that during the examination the healer should make visual observations, such as a patient exhibiting shortness of breath, insatiable thirst or other symptoms not easily explainable. The healer might then push for a thorough urinalysis. It may prove fruitless in determining Bright's disease or Diabetes, but the healer's intuition would help guide treatment and ease the patient's mind to rule out these ailments. Lastly, the most important part of the diagnosis was the patient's mental state. At this point, the healer had to determine what he could cause the patient to think, different from how the patient already thought. The same held true for what the healer must cause the patient to do, different from what the patient already did. The rationale was that once the treatment was administered to an approved plan, the healer had impressed upon the patient to follow the healer's directions to the letter.

Weltmer cautioned the healer to be conservative in giving directions, but once it was determined to be essential, the healer had to see that they were carried out. Weltmer stated: "If the patient is to walk a half mile every morning before breakfast and the patient does not see fit to follow these directions, and after a brief and definite argument he does not agree to do it, it is then your duty to dismiss the case."[6]

Weltmer reiterated that the healer be very careful not to advise any special exercise until the healer was fully convinced that such exercises were necessary to the best interests of the patient. Another advantage with a thorough diagnosis was that the healer didn't need to ask the patient any further about his illness and, therefore, prohibited the patient from saying anything to the healer or anyone else until there was a good report to make. By following this format, it enabled the healer to reasonably impress every patient to not think of or discuss their condition. The best results were for the patient to not only "forget it," but make a conscious effort to keep his thoughts on pleasant and agreeable things, so that the treatment effect would remain as long as possible after each treatment.[7]

After Lizzie determined she could help the patient, she would recommend a treatment plan. Weltmer stressed that the healer should "not" take any case for less than six treatments. His rationale was that the healer needed a fair chance to make a cure and would require at least six treatments to do so.[8] He also maintained that healer needed to complete the patient-record card while it was fresh in the healer's mind and before treatments began.

To secure a treatment plan with the patient, Weltmer suggested having a "treatment ticket" on hand with the inducement of one free treatment when paying for six in advance. He concluded that the ticket nearly always made the sale and simplified cash collections, plus got the payment issue out of the way.

Weltmer Treatment Ticket ➡️

						Graduate of the Weltmer Institute of Suggestive Therapeutics
(Free) TREATMENTS	TREATMENTS	TREATMENTS	TREATMENTS	TREATMENTS	TREATMENT	PATIENT'S TREATMENT CARD NO. 57————
						ISSUED TO
						M————————————————————
						In charge of ————————————————
						Time———————— Date————————
						PAYMENT IN ADVANCE RECEIVED.
6	5	4	3	2	1	Per————————
						No. 105 s. t.

Lizzie's treatment tickets were distributed by color. Pink may have been the six paid in advance with one free. Green, pay-as-you-go with a discounted rate. Beige, miscellaneous at standard rate. Her cards were also used as appointment reminders, circling the month and days at the top and the bottom. It is unknown what Lizzie charged, but in Weltmer's *How to Succeed* book, published in 1912, he used $2.50[s] per treatment as an example.

S.L. SNYDER COLOR-CODED TREATMENT CARDS
(Author's collection)

---

[s] About $75 in today's money.

WELTMER PATIENT RECORD CARD (EXAMPLE)
National Archives
(The Weltmer Institute, 1919, *How to Succeed*)
(Public domain)

The patient's record card was a brief history and weekly report of progress. Each column represented a week. In the example of week two, the patient was B (better) and continued to improve (OK). By week three, he was pronounced well and discharged from treatment (circled above).

For potential patients, who had inquired about treatment but had not committed, Weltmer advised to gather as much information as possible and create a follow-up card. Below is an example from the *How to Succeed* book. If days went by without contact, Weltmer recommended follow-up letters.

HOW TO KEEP YOUR RECORDS.   59

| 1-2 | 3-5 | 6-8 | 9-11 | 12-13 | 14-16 | 17-18 | 19-21 | 22-23 | 24-26 | 27-28 | 29-31 | LIST |

NAME **Brown, Wm. J.** BUSINESS **(Farmer)** STATE **Mo.**

DATE	R. R. STR. OR BOX NO.		NATION	**P. T.**
June 7		Rural Route #2-Box 31		
1911	SOURCE of INQUIRY	Popular Therapeutics-June		DUPLICATE

LITERATURE SENT			FORM LETTERS		PAST PURCHASE CHRONOLOGICAL		
					Art'l.	Date	Am't
A		E	1	FU#1-6/11/11	Reg	7-5-11	$2.00
B		F	2	FU#2-6/21/11			
C		G	3	FU#3-7/21/11			
D		H	4				

DICTATED LETTERS, SPC'L. TERMS, REMARKS **Will return be-before 11th for exm.& tr.Judge Adams called on him, says he may come in few days-wants book to read on subject 7/11/11.A**

WELTMER FOLLOW-UP CARD
National Archives
(The Weltmer Institute, 1919, *How to Succeed*)
(Public domain)

When conducting business, Weltmer underscored that the patient's interest was always first, finances secondary:

> *If a party should come to you not able to pay or arrange for payment for your treatments, then treat that party free. Get in debt to no one in the community, if it can be avoided, and be sure and let no one get in debt to you.*[9]

He concluded that there was nothing worse than the trouble and criticism as the collection of bills. In the event that you treated a person and were unable to collect payment after two or three friendly reminders, send a final receipted bill with a note that the debt has been erased from your books.

SANIPRACTIC is the science and art of applied prophylactic and therapeutic sanitation, which enables the physician to direct, advise, prescribe or apply food water, roots, herbs, light, heat, exercise (passive and active), manipulation, adjusting tissue, vital organs or anatomical structure by manual, mechanical or electrical instruments or appliances; or other natural agency to assist nature restore a psychological and physiological interfunction for the purpose of maintaining a normal state of health in mind and body.

Copyright, 1919.

The American University of Sanipractic

1134 SEVENTEENTH AVENUE

(at E. Union St.)

Dr. S. L. Snyder,

Dear Doctor: Seattle, Wash., July 28, 1920.

      Opportunities come and go. They often depart unheeded and return no more. A great opportunity is now at your door.

      Dr. Gregory, the greatest author of rational therapy methods and the most successful teacher of Postgraduate Courses, who has gathered so much practical and helpful information since beginning his public lectures ten years ago, is now in Seattle and will conduct a special Postgraduate course beginning August 2nd, 8 p.m., at American University of Sanipractic, corner Seventeenth and East Union.

      Dr. Gregory is getting wonderful results by using his combined drugless methods, usually overcoming, with a single treatment, such diseases as appendicitis, angina pectoris, diarrhoea, diphtheria, "flu," pneumonia, scarlet fever, tic-dou-loureux, acute tonsilitis, lumbago and sciatica and other acute diseases.

THE AMERICAN UNIVERSITY OF SANIPRACTIC
Dr. Gregory Post-Graduate Course
(July 28, 1920)
(Author's collection)

12
ZONE THERAPY

AUGUST 1920, while staying with Etta and Lester, Lizzie attended the "American University of Sanipractic Post-Graduate course," taught by Dr. Gregory in Seattle. Dr. Gregory specialized in various drugless treatments for such diseases as Brights, inflammatory rheumatism, and the lowering of blood pressure from 240 to normal. He advertised that recent students were getting better results with three treatments than the previous ten with former methods.[1] It was during this trip that Lizzie began expanding her research on "Zone Therapy." Shortly after this visit, she added it as a treatment option.

ZONE THERAPY, developed by American physician William H. Fitzgerald, is the use of pressure points to relieve pain. A graduate of the University of Vermont, Dr. Fitzgerald worked at the Boston City Hospital, the Central London Nose and Throat Hospital, and later was the senior nose and throat surgeon of St. Francis Hospital in Hartford. During his early years, he was an assistant to Professors Politzer and Otto Chiari of Vienna, famous authors of medical textbooks.[2] Dr. Edwin F. Bowers, also an American physician, later joined Dr. Fitzgerald with his research.

Dr. Bowers described Dr. Fitzgerald as able, honest, and competent. He also stated that no matter how ridiculous his methods appeared, they were the calmly digested findings of a trained scientific mind. In 1917, the Drs. co-wrote the book: *Zone Therapy or Relieving Pain at Home.*

Zone therapy is divided into ten vertical zones that correspond to fingers and toes all the way up to the head. The diagram zones are numbered 1 through 5 on one side of the body, but are identical on both sides. Each number represents the center of its respective zone for the anterior and posterior views.[3]

The anterior zones include the tongue, hand, and generative organs. The middle ear, on both sides of the head, is in zone 4 of the soft palate, the nasopharynx and oropharynx, and the generative organs. The teeth, viscera, and tongue are located in both the anterior and the posterior zones. The upper tongue is in the anterior and the under surface, the posterior. The hand follows a similar format. The back, to the front of the body, and the palm, the sole of the foot.

Diagram A
Anterior Zone

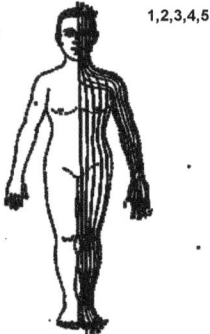

1,2,3,4,5

Diagram B
Posterior Zone

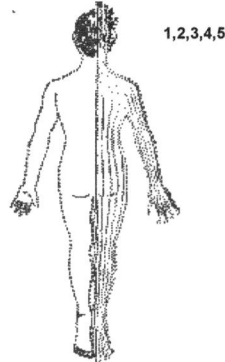

1,2,3,4,5

Diagrams A&B: *Zone Therapy for Relieving Pain at Home,* 1917
Wm H. Fitzgerald, M.D. and Edwin F. Bowers, M.D., 13-14
(Courtesy of University of California Libraries, B890-554z, 1917
A000 416 983 5)
All books published prior to 1927 are public domain

After Drs. Fitzgerald and Bowers lectured at the Riley School of Chiropractic in Washington D.C., Dr. Riley began using zone therapy on his patients with much success. He further expanded zone therapy by adding eight horizontal divisions of the feet and hands, which was the beginning of reflexology. His work also included the ears and other parts. During his lifetime, Dr. Riley wrote twelve books on the subject and traveled nationwide with his wife, Elizabeth Ann Riley, giving lectures and demonstrations including a technique called hook work, which was the manipulation of the fingers to aid in relief of pain to other areas of the body.

Specialist in zone therapy found that pressure was effective in deadening pain or making it more bearable in about 80% of cases. While there were no claims that zone pressure could cure cancer, there had been cases of tumor reduction and reports where the pain had been relieved and freed the patient from resorting to opiates.[4] Several of Lizzie's drawings and notes referenced Dr. Riley's name, but many of her sketches are from Drs. Fitzgerald and Bowers' book as well.

ONE CAN VISUALIZE Lizzie sitting at a table in the research library, books scattered across as she sketched diagrams and transcribed notes. Her notes correspond with her drawings, which were done in pen on vellum paper.

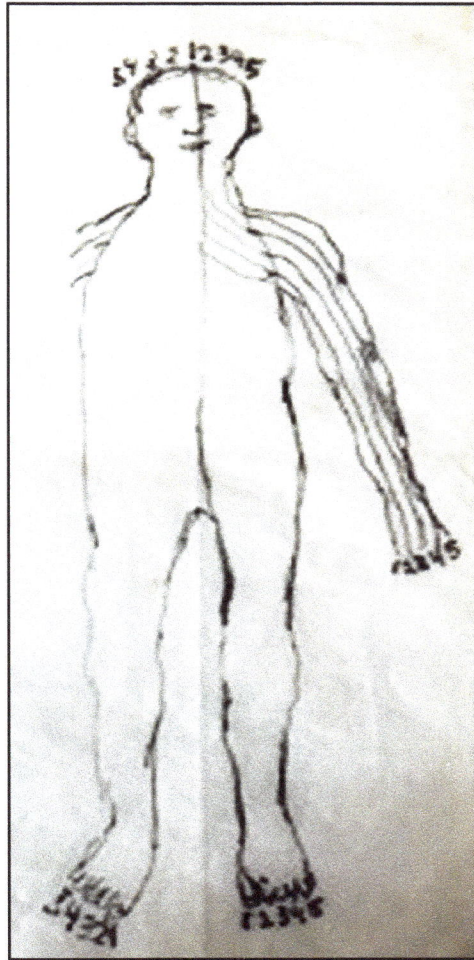

ANTERIOR ZONE
Drawn by Lizzie
1920
(Author's collection)

LIZZIE'S NOTES
Reference J.S. Riley's name at the top
(Author's collection)

Several of the treatments include the use of rubber bands, clothes pins, and special tools. Drs. Fitzgerald and Bowers' book, *Zone Therapy or Relieving Pain at Home,* 1917, provides multiple illustrations as featured on the following pages. One can only imagine a patient's reaction when Lizzie suggested putting clothespins or rubber bands on their fingers or a surgical clamp on their tongue.

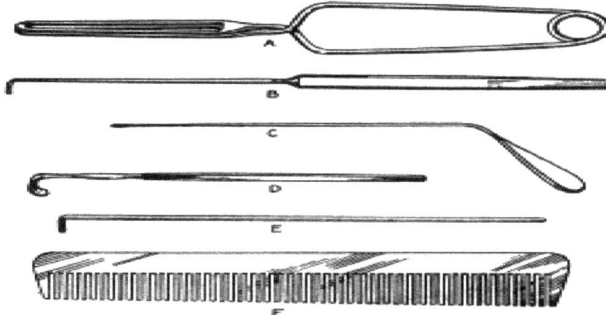

48 ZONE THERAPY.

Non-Electrical Applicators Useful in Zone Therapy

A is an ordinary surgical clamp which can be used for clamping the tongue.

B is an ordinary eye-muscle retractor. This can be used for intermittently retracting the posterior pillars of the fauces.

C is a special type of nasal probe used for attacking the posterior wall of the nasopharynx.

D is a regular palpebral retractor which can be used for intermittently retracting the soft palate, especially in the region of the fossa of Rosenmüller.

E is a regular flat applicator bent up at one end. This is useful about the throat and fauces. It can be used as a pressure applicator for the posterior wall of the oropharynx.

F is an ordinary aluminum comb used for attacking the fingers or toes either at the tips or about the joints.

FIG. 11.

Figure T1, page 48
Zone Therapy or Relieving Pain at Home, **Drs. Fitgerald & Browers (1917)**
(Courtesy of Library of Congress, Internet Archive Open Library)
(Public domain)

- Surgical clamp for clamping the tongue.
- Eye-muscle retractor (forceps) for retracting posterior pillars of the fauces.[t]
- Nasal probe for attacking the posterior wall of nasopharynx.
- Palpebral retractor for retracting soft palate.
- Flat applicator bent up at one end for throat and fauces. It was also used for the posterior wall of the oropharynx.
- Aluminum comb for attacking fingers and toes at the tips or about the joints.

---

[t] Fauces: the arched opening at the back of the mouth to the pharynx between the soft palate and base of the tongue.

Hollowed-out spring clothespins are used for the relief of pain and to desensitize the teeth for dental procedures. Also touted as the most effective cure for an earache is placing the clothespin at the tip of the ring finger for five minutes.

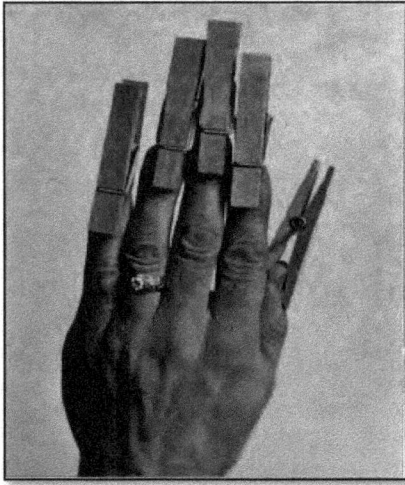

Figure 13, page 59
*Zone Therapy or Relieving
Pain at Home,* 1917

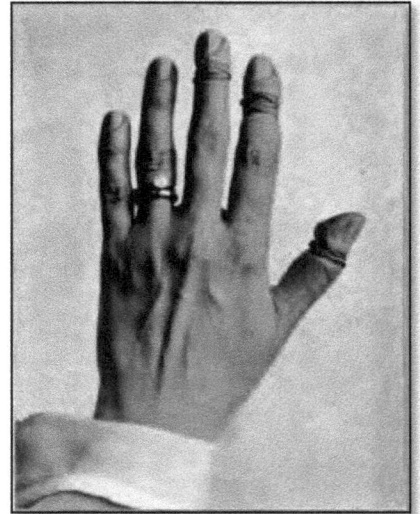

Rubber bands are used for treatments of deafness, bladder pains, and the lowering of blood pressure by placing the rubber bands around the fingers or toes for a few minutes, two or three times a day.

Figure 5, page 22
*Zone Therapy or Relieving
Pain at Home,* 1917

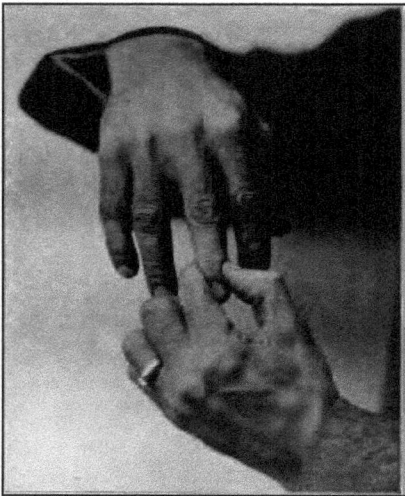

Squeezing the side of the fingers also relieves pain.

Figure 4, page 20
*Zone Therapy or Relieving
Pain at Home,* 1917

The aluminum comb is used for various treatments, such as: deafness, lumbago and pains in the back of the body. Pressure on the finger tips affect both the anterior and posterior in the 2nd, 3rd, 4th, and 5th zones.

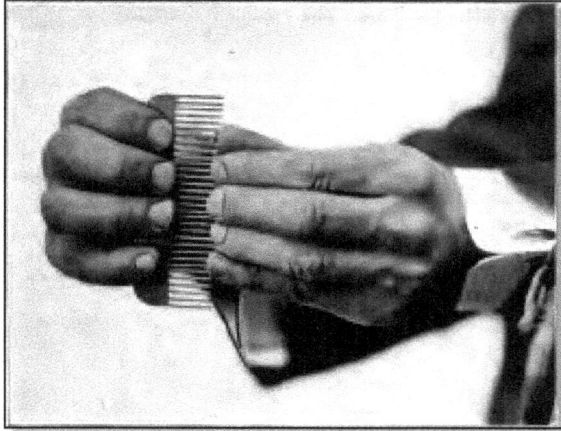

Figure 12, page 55
*Zone Therapy or Relieving
Pain at Home,* 1917

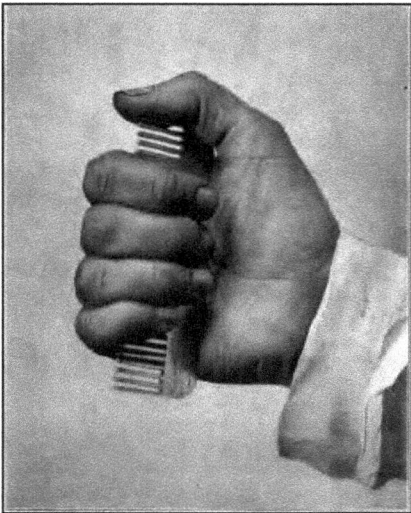

Figure 14, page 63
*Zone Therapy or Relieving
Pain at Home,* 1917

Lizzie's sketches from the pictures in the zone-therapy books.

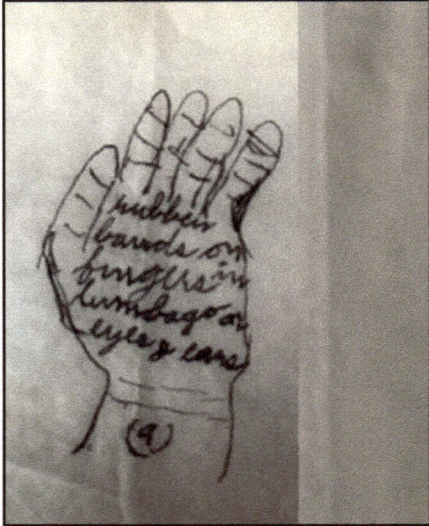

Rubber bands

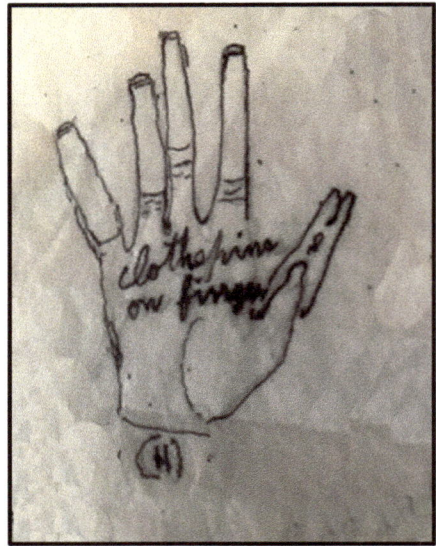

Clothespins

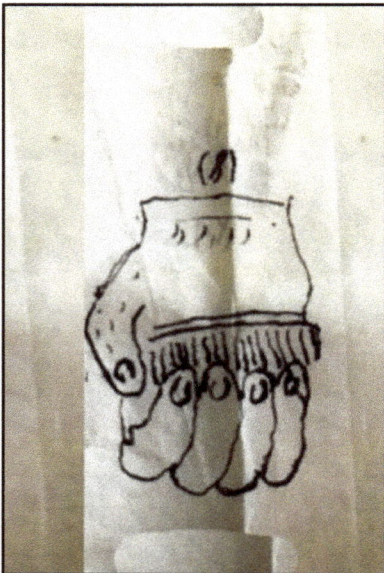

Aluminum Comb

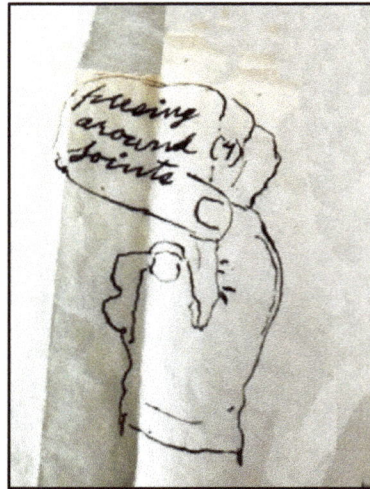

Pressing outside finger joints

LIZZIE'S ZONE-THERAPY DRAWINGS
S.L. Snyder Artifacts
(Author's collection)

No. 3, Nervousness Zone: Sciatic rheumatism, diabetics, painful childbirth, stomach ulcer, and blood pressure. The treatments vary with the use of the aluminum comb, clothespins, rubber bands, and a mallet. Lizzie's drawings accompany ten pages of detailed notes.

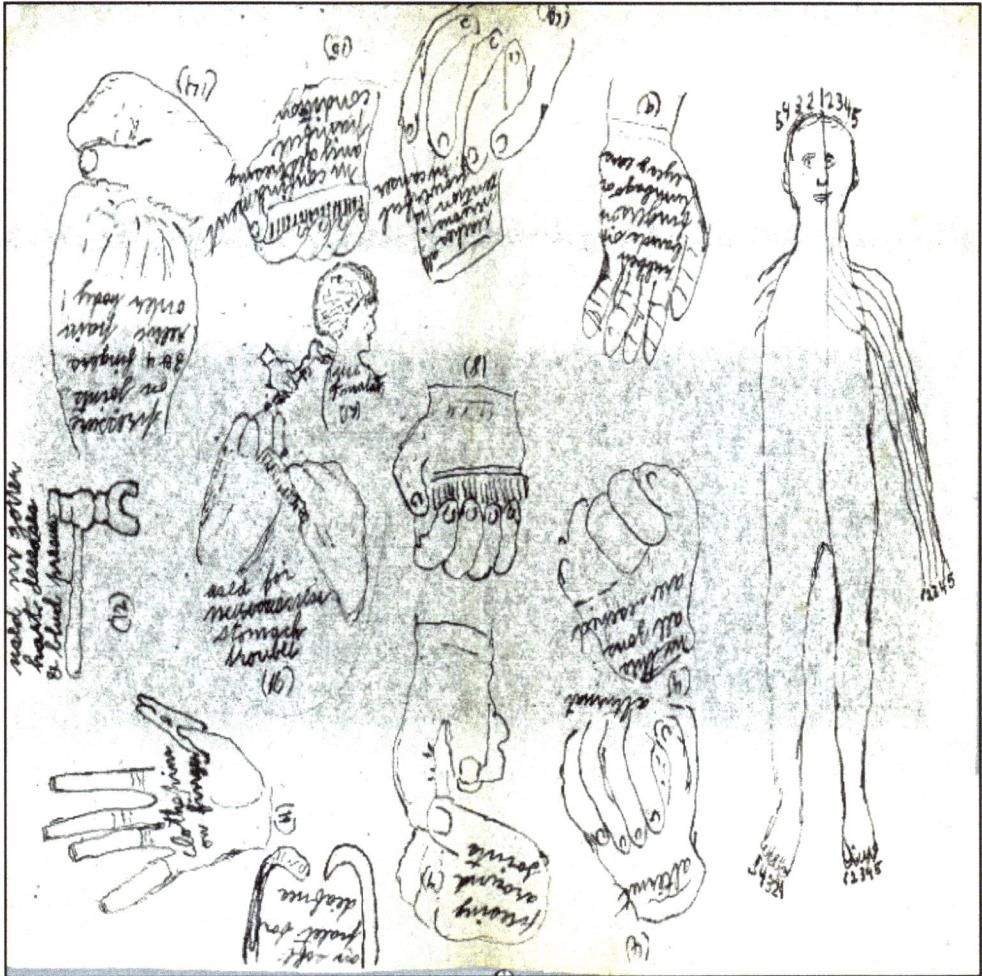

LIZZIE'S ZONE-THERAPY DRAWINGS
(Author's collection)

LIZZIE'S NOTES
(Author's collection)

No. 3: Nervousness Zone:

Use aluminum comb or good stiff brush over backs and fronts of fingers for 5 to 7 minutes. Press firmly finger tips about same length of time. Pressure on toungue [sic] a few minutes each day. Clothespins on fingers will bring equally good results. Nervousness, sleeplessness be overcome by pressing teeth firmly together. Also interlacing fingers firmly together.

13
CONCLUSION

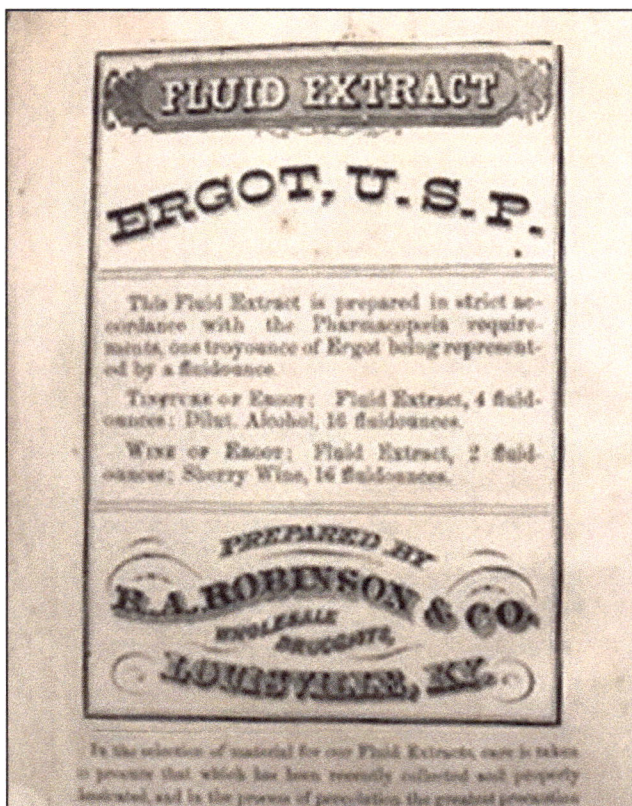

LIZZIE'S FORMULARY BOOK
(Author's collection)

ERGOT has been used for centuries by midwives, but with care due to toxicity. In the 20th century, scientists isolated specific ergot alkaloids and turned them into drugs. Ergotamine today is a treatment for migraines and used by doctors in precise doses to prevent bleeding after birth. Ergot-based medications are currently being researched for Parkinson's disease and dementia.[1]

After the rise of the suffragette movement in the late nineteenth century, women gradually gained acceptance into medical schools. Many of these new doctors embraced the new theories of natural cures, hygiene, and preventative medicine, but to avoid further ridicule from their male counterparts, they were urged to follow the scientific orthodox treatments instead.[2] One of the treatments included bloodletting either by a physician or by leeches.

Elizabeth Blackwell, the first American Physician to earn a medical degree on January 23, 1849, recalled the horror of witnessing how brutally male doctors treated female gynecological examinations. As a result, she was determined even more to become a doctor so that women could be treated by a member of their own sex.[3] When she did open her own practice in New York, she faced vast opposition from men within the medical profession and those not associated at all. After a series of lectures on physical education for girls with handouts, she founded a small dispensary for working-class women and their children. She later opened a medical college for women and added natural medicines and hygiene to the curriculum. She fought for similar changes in England.

By the early twentieth century when Lizzie entered the healing field (1901), women practitioners were few and far between. The suppression of female healers had been a political struggle. They were first attacked because they were "women," secondly because of their "class." Women healers were the people's doctors and their medicine a part of a people's subculture. For centuries, the wise woman or witch, which they were often called, had a host of remedies used in modern medicine today. Throughout history, it was women who were the independent healer and often the only healers for the women and the poor. [4] Women frequently went into joint practices with their husbands. The husband handled the surgery, the wife, midwifery, gynecology, and everything else shared.[5]

It is known that Lizzie used midwives with all of her childbirths as referenced in Florence's 1962 letter, stating that she had been born in the Hoquiam boardinghouse. Many women were not comfortable going to male doctors. Women practitioners were also viewed as more sympathetic and better listeners,[6] and having someone like Lizzie calmed their concerns. The majority of Lizzie's patients were women, but she did not perform midwifery herself, instead she instructed and treated women-related ailments and was at the birth if the patient requested her presence. She had books specific to women's health and remedies from her formulary book, such as Ergot used for uterine problems and for possible problematic childbirth deliveries. She also had extensive women-related treatments outlined in her zone-therapy notes, which included fibroid tumors, menstruation, pregnancy, and childbirth.

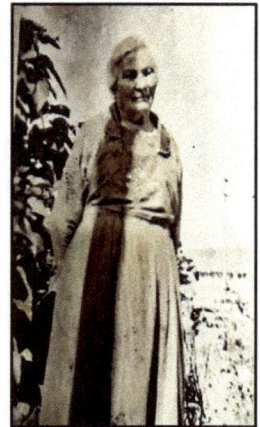

Auntie Girard, Midwife. Delivered Florence Snyder 1898.
(Author's collection)

Same as many of the women practitioners before her, Lizzie pressed for preventative measures such as proper diet, sleep, and exercise. In most cases, it was more of an afterthought as most of her patients only appeared if they were ill, but one can hope that her power of persuasion changed their direction.

While still performing their duties, women healers of the past had to be silent, careful and at the same time outspoken.[7] Many times nothing was documented, only passed down from a wise woman to a daughter or a niece or trusted female who showed healing promise.

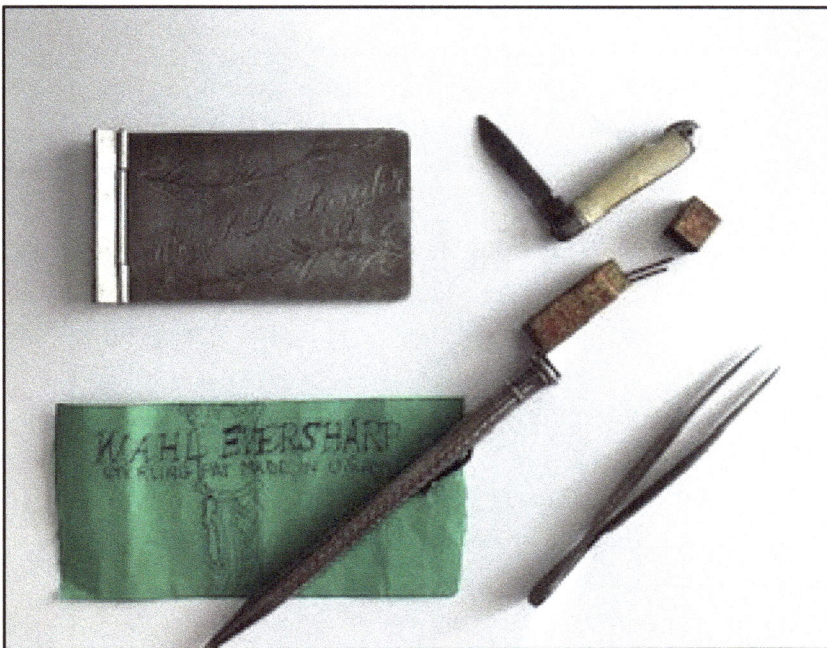

Items used by S.L. Snyder in her healing practice.
(Author's collection)

- Tweezers
- Pen knife
- Pencil (Wahl Eversharp-Sterling U.S.A)
- Pencil Box with refills
- Metal card holder (Engraved: Mrs. S.L. Snyder)

AFTER TWENTY-SEVEN YEARS as a healer, Lizzie officially closed her practice in 1928. Partly because the sanipractic and other drugless professions were under attack by the medical community. The loss of her grandson, Herman, Lester and Etta's child, also affected her.

Physicians across the states began lobbying for new laws requiring license applicants to pass examinations in anatomy, physiology, pathology, and other science basics before taking their licensing test in their special system of therapy. In 1925, Wisconsin was the first to pass the act into law, followed by twenty-three states.[8] The two years preceding the 1927 statue, there were more chiropractors licensed in Washington State than MDs (forty-seven doctors, forty-eight chiropractors, forty-four sanipractors, *one of those Lizzie*, and thirty-eight osteopaths. By 1929, the medical doctors grew to eighty, but only six osteopaths, one chiropractor, and no drugless healers remained.[9]

Many of the drugless healers weren't equipped educationally to take the science exam, but others, like Lizzie, who had been educated in these studies, had grown tired of the ridicule. They were being referred to as cultist, intellectually inferior, and their treatments a form of voodoo mixed with snake oil, plus touted as money-grabbers. This is not to say that the medical profession didn't have some merit to their claims. Even progressives within naturopathy were outspoken over the infiltration by charlatans looking for easy money.

Between the late 1920's and early 1930's, all states with boards had a basic-science exam with a success rate of ninety percent for physicians, sixty-three percent for osteopaths, and twenty-seven percent for chiropractors. As time passed, the medical profession discovered that the laws they had pushed to pass had backfired. Osteopathic, chiropractic, and other drugless schools had elevated their training to include medical science. Weltmer Institute had already proceeded down this path years prior, so when Lizzie attended she had received much of the necessary training. With slow, steady improvement in the passing rates, the basic-science exams became less effective in separating what the medical field viewed as *cultist* from the scientist. The most rapid progress was achieved by osteopathy.

In the years 1942 through 1953, the basic-science exams shot up from fifty-two percent to eighty percent (physicians' rate was eighty-seven).[10] Today, many of the treatments that Lizzie and her father performed are still viable, such as hypnosis used in psychotherapy.[11] Mechano-therapy, in Lizzie and Professor Wilson's practice, was a form of chiropractic. Electrotherapy, the modern-day TENS machine. Hydrotherapy is one of many physical-therapy treatments. Zone therapy expanded into reflexology. Herbs and spices listed in her formulary book are still used today, such as Arrowroot, which is gluten-free and contains more fiber than potatoes as well as a good amount of potassium, iron, and vitamin B's. It is also known to stimulate the immune system and treat diarrhea.

Suggestive Therapeutics can be viewed in many terms, maybe as simple as positive affirmation to a patient or by the patient themselves to aid in their healing. And Weltmer's philosophy that God was Law. Many with serious illnesses have persevered beyond what modern medicine could do and survived with no reasonable explanation, except for one—a *miracle.*

Lizzie and her father helped many in need. Her father's untimely death ended his practice, but prior to his passing, he was still enhancing his skills. Lizzie initially followed his healing guidance, but she expanded into so much more.

Being born blind hindered her learning, even basic reading and math skills, these came later with her mother's help and instruction. But it put a spark in Lizzie to want to know more and not let obstacles hold her back. Approaching forty, she stepped into the healing role.

Several of her research books from the early 1900's endorsed healthy eating, exercise, and proper sleep, and continue as the current view. Even fasting may have seemed far-fetched but a proven theory today. She believed in what she was doing and strived to be the best she could be. I, KB Taylor, her great-granddaughter, am so grateful that I happened upon my cousin's home that day. Not only were Lizzie's artifacts worth saving, but as I unraveled her story, they provided one worth telling and allowed me the opportunity to know a remarkable woman.

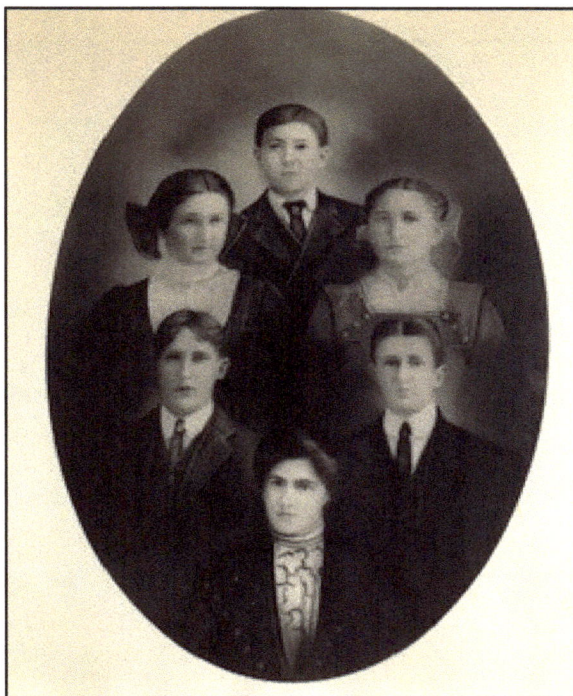

LIZZIE'S CHILDREN

Front: Mary Belle Rodgers
Middle (L to R)   William Jr. and Lester Hanson
Back: (L to R)   Jessie, Lincoln, Florence Snyder

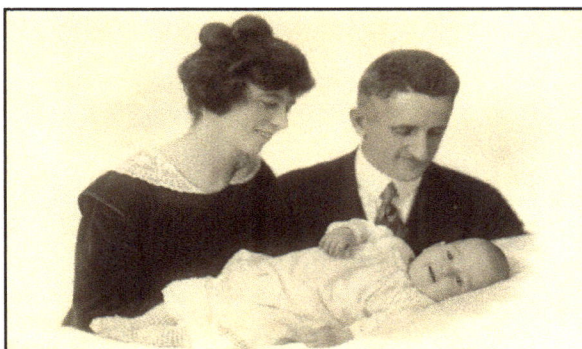

ETTA AND LESTER HANSON
with firstborn, Herman
(Author's collection)

145

My mother was a Saniprodic & Chiroproctor physician. The class of 1918 was the first class to go through the last four grade in the new high school. I graduated in 1918.

Florence Oviatt

LAST PAGE OF FLORENCE SNYDER'S 1962 LETTER
(Author's collection)

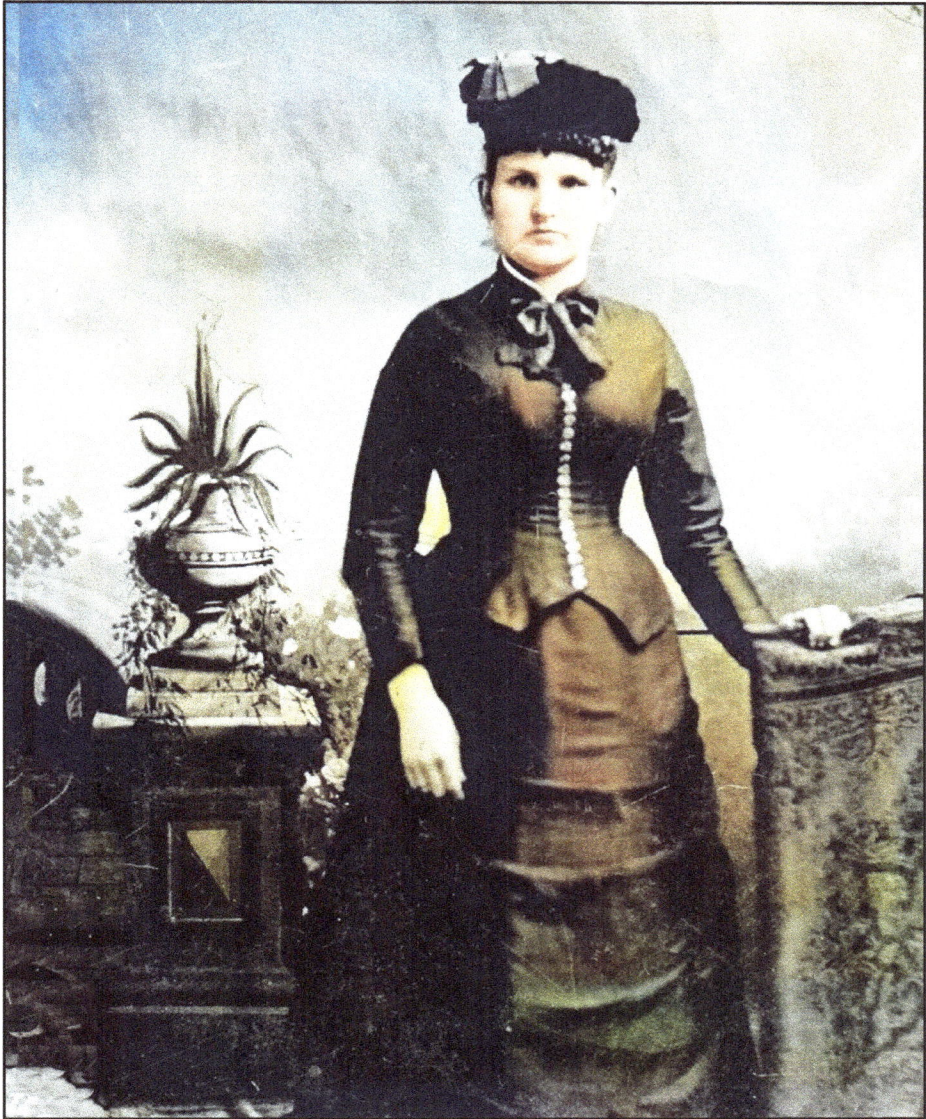

S.L. SNYDER (LIZZIE)
Sanipractic Physician

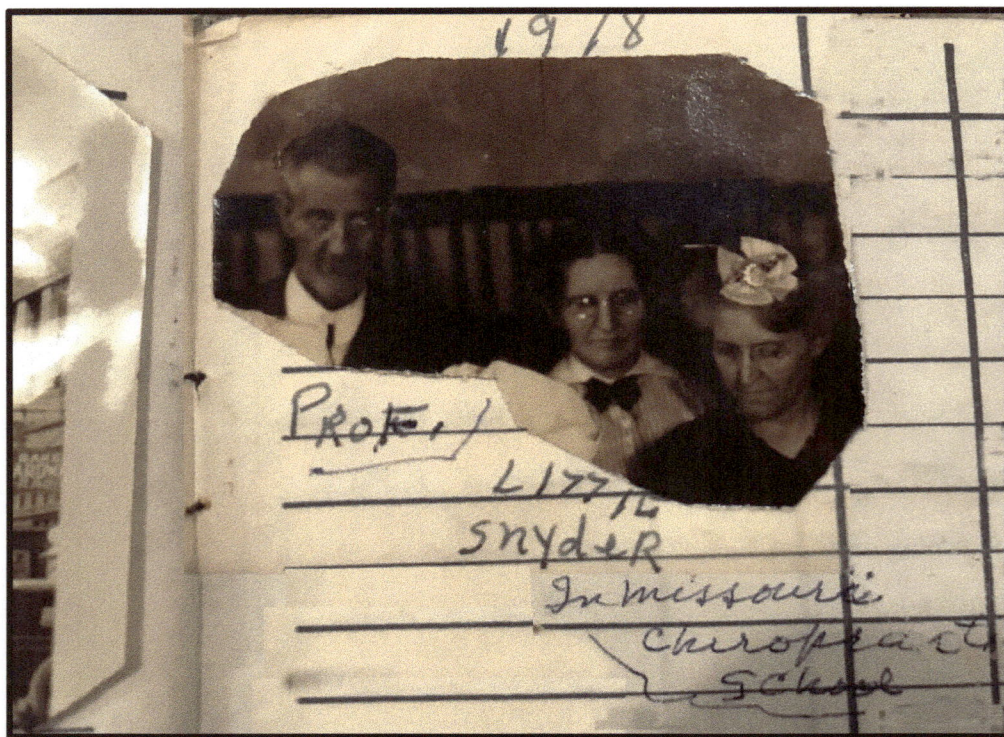

**LIZZIE SNYDER WITH A "WELTMER PROFESSOR" AND
FELLOW STUDENT AT THE "WELTMER INSTITUTE,"
MISSOURI**
Top portion is Lizzie's handwriting

Description was later added by her daughter, Florence.
Florence always referred to the "Weltmer Institute" as a
Chiropractic School

NOTES

Introduction

1 *The Hamburg Reporter*, March 1911. Find a Grave, Memorial #23082182:

> *Andrew Jackson WILSON, b. in Greene county, Ohio - died at his home in Hamburg on Mar. 22, 1911 aged 95 years 5 months. Came to Fremont county as a young man and was one of the pioneers of Fremont county.* **In Mr. Wilson's early days he became a strong abolitionist, and in 1847 was a conductor on the underground railway at Oskaloosa, Iowa, where it is authoritatively stated he assisted many negroes to escape. He read "Uncle Tom's Cabin" as it appeared in the Liberator, previous to the time it was published in book form.....**He *resided four miles north of Hamburg in what was first Holt county, Missouri, and later Atchison county, Missouri, and later with the establishment of the Mason and Dixon line, it became Pottawattamic county, Mills county and later Fremont county, Iowa. In 1869 Mr. Wilson removed to Hamburg where he has since resided. Note: After his first wife died in 1872, he later married secondly to a lady named Mary McDaniel Hamilton in 1874. Her husband J. William Hamilton died Feb 10, 1874.*

2 Aberdeen History, historylink.org.
3 *Women in White Coats*, Park Row Books, 2021, Olivia Campbell, 12.
4 Ibid, 13.
1 Viorene **Gladys** (née May) Muhlhauser's documentation (Florence Snyder's daughter). **(Hereafter GM documentation.)**
2 Pension Affidavit to U.S. Department of Interior 1898, Mattie McClure (William B. Wilson's sister). See Affidavit, page 156.
3 GM documentation.
4 *The River Pioneers: Early Days on Grays Harbor* by Edwin Van Syckle, 193, 1982.
5 GM documentation.

Chapter Two—The Boardinghouse

1 www.history.com/Chinese Immigration in America
2 *The River Pioneers, Early Days on Grays Harbor* by Edwin Van Syckle, 379, 1982. "Eviction of the Chinese."
3 Ibid.
4 GM documentation.
5 *Arequipa Sanatorium, Life in California's Lung Resort for Women*, Lynn Downey, University Press, 2019, 53.
6 Ibid, 52.
7 www.history.com/news/midterm-elections-biggest-landslide- Republicans-Grover-Cleveland.
8 *The Panic of 1893: The Untold Story of Washington State's First Depression,* Bruce A. Ramsey, 2018.
9 Ibid.
10 J. Snyder Nov.1894 letter to Lizzie. See letter, page 160.

Chapter Three—Weltmer

[1] *The Kansas City Journal*, July 1899, Weltmer Ad, enlarged copy, page 161.

[2] *Missouri Historical Review,* "Weltmer, Stanhope, and the Rest , Magnetic Healing in Nevada Nevada, Missouri" by Patrick Brophy, 275-294, April 1997. (Courtesy of the Bushwhacker Museum, Nevada, Mo.).

[3] Ibid, 279.

[4] Ibid, 279.

[5] Ibid, 277.

[6] *Mystery Revealed* by S.A. Weltmer, published 1901, digital collection, public domain, 7-8.

[7] Ibid, 8.

[8] Ibid, 10.

[9] Ibid, 113.

[10] Ibid, 114-116.

[11] Ibid, 119-123.

[12] *Missouri Historical Review;* "Weltmer, Stanhope, and the Rest: Magnetic Healing in Nevada, Mo." by Patrick Brophy, April 1997,289.(Courtesy of the Bushwhacker Museum, Nevada, Mo.)

[13] *Mystery Revealed* by S.A. Weltmer, published 1901, public domain,178, Hypnotism.

[14] Ibid, 147, 148, Heating the Hands.

[15] Ibid, 64-66, Agreement.

[16] *The Healing Hand*, by S.A. Weltmer, published 1922, public domain, 177, Home Treatment Service.

[17] Ibid, 177.

[18] *Missouri Historical Review;* "Weltmer,Stanhope, and the Rest: Magnetic Healing in Nevada, Missouri" by Patrick Brophy, April 1997, 293 (William S. Brink, letter 10 September 1984) (Courtesy of the Bushwhacker Museum, Nevada, Mo.)

[19] Ibid, 292.

[20] Ibid; *Nevada Daily Mail*, April 7, 2017, Carolyn Gray Thornton.

[21] *Telepathy: Its Theory, Facts and Proof* by William Walker Atkinson, published 1910.

[22] "Tri-County Genealogical Society, Nevada, Mo., August 8, 2008 Newsletter."

[23] *Missouri Historical Review;* "Weltmer, Stanhope, and the Rest: Magnetic Healing in Nevada, Missouri" by Patrick Brophy, April 1997, 279. (Courtesy of Bushwhacker Museum, Nev., Mo.)

[24] *Pioneer Teachers*, F.H. Behncke, Published 1920, Phineas Parkhurst Quimby, 70.

[25] www.newthoughtwisdom.com/about-new-thought-html.

[26] John Bruno Hare, Internet Sacred Text archive; www.sacred-Texts.com.

[27] Britannica.com/event/New-Thought.

[28] *Mystery Revealed* by S.A. Weltmer, published 1901, public domain, 6; *Weltmerism*, Chapter1.

[29] *Rediscover Nevada, Mo!* February 12, 2008.

[30] *Missouri Historical Review;* "Weltmer, Stanhope, and the Rest: Magnetic Healing in Nevada, Missouri" by Patrick Brophy, April 1997, 291, 292 (Robert Lowell Stone, Jr., "Weltmer: Pioneer of Psychotherapy.") (Courtesy of the Bushwhacker Museum, Nevada, Mo.)

Chapter Four—Weltmer Institute

[1] *Nevada Daily Mail*, January 13, 1900. (Bushwhacker Museum archives, Nevada, Mo.)

[2] *Weltmerism* magazine, April 1901, 9

[3] **Weltmer Resident Course**, State Historical Society of Missouri (SHSMO) artifact. (Courtesy of the Bushwhacker Museum, Nevada, Mo.) Document, see page 162.

Chapter Five—93 Market Street

[1] *How to Succeed/Weltmer*, 17 (Rules). Published 1912. The Weltmer Institute of Suggestive Therapeutics Company, Nevada, Mo, National Archives, digitized, public domain.

[2] Ibid, 181.

[3] Weltmer, plate 2 caption. (Courtesy of the Bushwhacker Museum, Nevada, Mo.)

[4] *The Mystery Revealed*, 177-182.

[5] Ibid, 147.

[6] Ibid, 137.

[7] Matthew 18:19, Amplified Bible, Classic Edition.

[8] *The Mystery Revealed,* Treatment In General,147.

[9] The Weltmer Method of Magnetic Healing, 1897, S.A. Weltmer, Letter No 8, Mental Science. (Prof. W.B. Wilson collection, Power of Suggestion).

[10] *The Healing Hand,* Positive and Passive Conditions,118-122.

[11] *Weltmerism* magazine, Nov 1900, 24.(Courtesy of the Bushwhacker Museum, Nevada, Mo.)

[12] *How to Succeed*/Weltmer, 13.

[13] Ibid, 14.

[14] Mary Wilson's 1903 letter to Lizzie. See letter, page 163.

Chapter Six—Hoquiam

[1] *Pioneer Teachers* by F.H. Behncke, published 1920, Andrew Tyler Still, 61.

[2] *Nature Cures: The History of Alternative Medicine in America* by James C. Whorton, Ph.D., Oxford University Press, 2002, 142-143.

[3] Ibid, 146-150,151.

[4] *Pioneer Teachers* by F.H. Behncke, published 1920, Andrew Tyler Still, 61-62.

[5] *Nature Cures: The History of Alternative Medicine in America* by James C. Whorton, Ph.D., Oxford University Press, 2002, 156.

Chapter Seven—On Her Own

[1] *Missouri Historical Review,* "Weltmer, Stanhope, and the Rest: Magnetic Healing in Nevada Missouri" by Patrick Brophy, 291; Robert L. Stone Jr., "Weltmer." (Bushwhacker Museum.)

[2] *Regeneration* by Weltmer, 1908, 134 (Author's copy.)

[3] *School Day's 1900*, Dedicated to the people of Hoquiam, Clara Knack Dooley, 1970 handwritten journal of childhood on the Queets River and Hoquiam; Hoquiam and Aberdeen, WA libraries, 9. (Author's copy.)

Chapter Eight—New Horizons

[1] Weltmer four-year-course pamphlet, 9.

[2] Suggestotherapy pamphlet.

[3] "For Permanent Health," 1913-1914 Weltmer bulletin (Bushwhacker Museum, Nevada, Mo.)

[4] Ibid.

Chapter Nine—Weltmer Institute

[1] Weltmer, September 1, 1909 form letter. (Courtesy of the Bushwhacker Museum, Nevada, Mo.)

[2] Weltmer four-year-course pamphlet. (Courtesy of the Bushwhacker Museum, Nevada, Mo.)

[3] Ibid, Synopsis of the Course Instruction, 15-21.

[4] *Women in White Coats*, 188.

[5] Ibid, 188.

[6] Ibid, 29-30.

[7] Weltmer four-year-course, Synopsis of the Course Instruction, Physiology,18.(Courtesy of the Bushwhacker Museum, Nevada, Mo.)

[8] *How to Succeed*/The Weltmer Institute,1912, 144.

[9] Ibid, 93-94.

Chapter Ten—Lizzie's Return

1   Lester's Letter, May 1918. See original letter, page 164
2   Return message to Lester, inside Mother's Day Card. See original letter, page 165.
3   University of Michigan Center for the History of Medicine; University of Michigan Library "Seattle 1918 Flu."
4   Polson Museum, Harbor History Highlight, "Grippe Hits Home: The 1918 Influenza Pandemic on Grays Harbor," John Larson, Museum Director, July 2020.
5   Ibid.
6   GM documentation.
7   *Witches, Midwives & Nurses: A History of Women Healers* by Barbara Ehrenreich/Deirdre English, Feminist Press, NY, 2010, 47.
8   The Ojibwe Native Americans/https://ojibwenativeamericans.weebly.com.
9   University of Michigan Center for the History of Medicine; University of Michigan Library "Seattle 1918 Flu."

Chapter Eleven—Sanipractic

1   *Nature Cures: The History of Alternative Medicine in America* by James C. Whorton, Ph.D., Oxford University Press, 2002, 192.
2   Ibid,194-195.
3   Ibid, 214.
4   American Association of United Drugless Physicians Convention, letter, page 166.
5   *How to Succeed*/The Weltmer Institute,1912, 66
6   Ibid, 72-73.
7   Ibid, 74.
8   Ibid, 64-65.
9   Ibid, 86.

Chapter Twelve—Zone Therapy

1   The American University of Sanipractic, Dr. Gregory post-graduate course, letter, page 167.
2   *Zone Therapy or Relieving Pain at Home* by Wm. H. Fritgerald, M.D. and Edwin F. Bowers, M.D., 1917, 9-10 (Courtesy of University of California) Internet Archive—All books published prior to 1927, public domain/*Pioneer Teachers*, F.H. Behncke, Zone Therapy, 65.
3   Ibid, 13 & 14.
4   Ibid, 17-21.

Chapter Thirteen—Conclusion

1   www.medicalnewstoday.com/articles/ergot_poisioning#ergot-medicine.
2   *Woman Healers: Portraits of Herbalist, Physicians, and Midwives* by Elisabeth Brooke, 1995, 94-95.
3   Ibid,98.
4   *Witches, Midwives & Nurses* by Barbara Ehrenreich & Dierdre English, Feminist Press, NY, 2010, 27-29.
5   Ibid, 65.
6   *Woman Healers: Portraits of Herbalist, Physicians, and Midwives* by Elisabeth Brooke,1995, 96.
7   Ibid, 151.

8   *Nature Cures: The History of Alternative Medicine in America* by James C. Whorton, Ph.D., Oxford University Press, 2002, 231-232.

9   Ibid, 231.

10   Ibid, 223-233.

11   Ibid, 283.

ORIGINAL LETTERS/CORRESPONDENCE

W.B. Wilson Pension Request (1888)
Notarized Affidavit by Mattie A. McClure (W.B. Wilson's sister)
describing life in Holt, Missouri and W.B. Wilson's chronic colitis
(Author's collection)

Aberdeen, Wash.
Oct 4th 1893.

Dear sister Lizzie;

We received your letter nearly two weeks ago.

No papa hasn't got me a saddle yet, and I don't want him to for I wouldn't ride on Topsy for anything. That fellow never sent his picture nor ever a ...

My short hand writing has gone up the flu... Papa and the boys have been hauling in wood. Frank was sick Monday night; had a pain in both sides.

Fred is cutting down a tree back of the house ...

Josie Wilson's letter, Oct 4,1893, Page 1
(Author's collection)

Josie Wilson's letter, Oct 4,1893, Page 2
"Mama is teaching Belle how to knit."
(Author's collection)

Hoquiam Wash July 10 1894

Lizzie Rogers:

My dear Lizzie;

I received your letter before the Fourth and was pleased to here from you again I am Sorry that you have So poor Place too Work. I would be very mutch pleased to have been with you on your vacation I know we would enjoy it. the reason I did not write Soon I was waiting for pay day to find out if I had enough money to Spair to send you to come over but I was disapointed. But next pay day look out for a fire if the Mill do not Shut down on the account of the Strike. I Suppose there is excitable times in Tacoma. We cant get the Mail half the time. But every body is exited over the Strike. I Suppose you are too. Your boys are Well, and every body else. We held quite a time here on the Fourth There was a large Crod and every thing went off Smoothly. The Workman had a dance but I did not go. Mrs Jewell is Nursing

John Snyder's July 10, 1894 Letter to Lizzie
(Author's collection)

157

This is to certify that Mrs. was born in July 15-1863, in the new of the Moon sign was in breast, Your nature is sympathetic. love of nature, of good ideas of duty, a lover of home, and its surroundings, An ideal companion, Kind and affectionate to family, a good financier, can if no dictation amass a small fortune, You have passed good opportunitys by neglect, You are well provided with electricity, The gift of the power of authority in you is more than an average, well qualified to make all happy that is around you, your council is good, and your decision is good, and can be taken for granted, You are sometimes too superstitious, sometimes too much self, in company you attention attetion and a good degree of Modification a word that you drop or utter has its firmness, you are the center of affection by your family, congenial near by to your childrens entreaties, a Kind Mother, good house Keeper, you may have had longing to become what you have tried and failed to become, you have had experiences you could not understand, powers you were afraid to speak about, you wonder why the health, you so sadly want is withheld from you, you may have longed and striven for earnestly for happiness, and yet have failed to find it, you may have fought serious battles to overcome poverty, and disaster, without a sign of success, it can be given to you the cause and cure of that state that makes poverty the initial step to the attainment of prosperity, it can be made plain to you, and will uncover the highest and best within you, you never have grasped the privilige that belongs to you, This power is implanted in you, a noble purp

John Snyder's November 1894 Letter to Lizzie
(Author's collection)

VIVID BLUE IS THE SUN

TINTS OF HEAVENLY BODIES NOT WHAT THEY SEEM.

Atmospheric Envelope Gives Distorted Colors to Celestial Luminaries—Sky Is Really Black, Says Prof. Langley.

From an Exchange.

"There can be no doubt of the correctness of Professor Langley's opinion that the sun is really blue and not yellow, as we see it," said Professor T. J. J. See, of the naval observatory at Washington, who has made himself famous recently as the discoverer of "double stars" in numbers hitherto undreamed of.

"You have only to imagine the atmospheric envelope of the earth, which hinders vision, removed, and the heavens are revealed to the eye in an altogether new and unfamiliar aspect. The sky in broad daylight is black, and the moon, if above the horizon, is no longer yellow but a brilliant white. Though the blue sun shines above, the stars are much brighter and more distinctly seen than ever before on the clearest night. Furthermore, they differ much in color, some of them being red, others blue, others rose color, others violet and yet others green.

"A strange aspect of the universe this would seem to be; and yet such is its true appearance, whereas we are accustomed to behold it altered to the eye by the interference of the atmosphere. As is well known, the sky looks blue because of the breaking up of the light by innumerable particles of dust and moisture afloat in the air. Take away this hindrance to vision and no longer will diffusion of sunlight obscure the view of the stars, each of which will shine like a separate lamp in the blackness of space.

All Stars Are Suns.

"The blue sun, under present circumstances, looks yellow because the blue light rays, having short wave lengths, do not easily penetrate the atmospheric coat of the earth. The yellow waves are much longer, and have a better chance to get through, hence the sun is yellow and sunlight is yellow.

"Now, as to the differing tints of the stars, we must understand that they vary in this respect with their age. To begin with, it is necessary to realize that, barring the moon and a few planets, of our own system, visible because they are near, all of the celestial bodies one sees in the heavens at night are suns—many of them hundreds of times as big as our own sun. The so-called milky way is a congress of suns, in which our orb of day is a rather inferior luminary.

"Planets in general, being dark and extinguished bodies, could not possibly be visible by their own light, and so we must perceive that every star which twinkles in the vault above us at night is a sun. By the aid of powerful telescope I have discovered about a dozen stars that are actually made visible by the reflected light of the suns about which they revolve, but they do not importantly concern the general proposition.

Tint Depends on Heat.

"The color of a star—otherwise to be termed a distant sun—varies according to its age. In its youth it is yellow; in its old age blue. The tint is a matter of temperature; the hotter a star, the bluer it gets, because great heat means an activity that engenders blue light waves. Sirius is a blue star, as seen through the telescopes, simply because it is so hot. Probably Sirius gives 100 times as much light as our sun, though it is only three, or, perhaps, four, times as big. Vega, in the constellation Lyra, hundreds of times as big as our sun, is blue, and the inference is that the heat it emits is tremendous.

"I have been speaking of the appearance of these stars as viewed through the medium of our atmosphere. Their colors, in some cases, are so vivid as to exhibit marked differences; but if the air envelope of the earth were taken away their varying tints would be much more noticeable. From what I have said you will have understood that the sums of the universe go through progressive alterations of hue as they grow older. Our own sun is becoming steadily bluer, because it is growing hotter. Every star, or sun, grows hotter and hotter up to a certain point in its history, and then cools. Our sun, through the contraction of its gaseous body, is still gaining temperature, while losing bulk at the rate of ten inches in diameter per diem. It will be ten inches

in an electric lamp. 'When,' as a famous astronomer says, 'we remember that the entire surface of the huge luminary is coated with these clouds, every particle of which is thus intensely luminous, we need no longer wonder at the dazzling brightness which, even across the awful gulf of 93,000,000 miles, produces for us the inconceivable glory of daylight.'

Will Utilize Solar Heat.

"The greatest and most important invention to be made in the next century will be a machine for storing the heat of the sun and transforming it into electricity or some other form suitable for ready employment. This heat, which is now permitted to go to waste, will be applied to the running of mills, the warming of houses, and every other purpose for which energy is utilized. It is worth mentioning in this connection that every square yard of the sun's surface emits an amount of heat equal to that of a blast furnace consuming one ton of coal every ten minutes. The heat given out by the solar globe in one second would raise 195,000,000 cubic miles of ice cold water to the boiling point, and of this heat the earth receives only one 2,000,000,000th part."

1,600 SORE ARMS.

At the Waldorf-Astoria. From Manager to Scullery Maid, All Have Been Vaccinated.

From the New York Journal.

It resembles bicycle face, and yet it is different. The guests of the Waldorf-Astoria have noticed that it is more acute. It afflicts every one of the 1,600 employes of the hotel from the manager down to the understudy of the acting deputy sub-assistant scullery maid.

They were all vaccinated on Friday and Saturday. The man who calls "Front" with the air of a satrap summoning his generalissimo wears an expression of sad preoccupation, and the boy in buttons who opens the main door for new arrivals ducks aside from the more impetuous ones for fear they should brush against his arm.

Mr. Boldt, the proprietor of the hotel, set a good example by offering his own arm to the lancet, and his is the only face in the hotel in which the apprehensiveness natural to a vaccinated person is lost beneath the irradiation springing from a duty nobly done.

Rank upon rank, corps after corps, the hotel servants were marshaled to the surgical office of the hotel. Dr. Calvin Adams, who lives and practices in the hotel, had the assistance of four colleagues, and they all worked hard. There may have been insurgent feelings in the breasts of some of the employes, but the order was peremptory, and they knew what refusal would mean.

The board of health took a paternal interest in this wholesale distribution of lymph where it would do the most good. The authorities are anxious that vaccination should be carried out systematically in large establishments, the homes of whose employes are scattered all over the city; and this applies especially to hotels, inasmuch as an outbreak of smallpox among a floating population might easily result in the spread of the disease far and wide before steps could be taken to confine it.

For these reasons all the employes of the Hotel Manhattan, Forty-second street and Madison avenue, were vaccinated a couple of weeks ago.

There was every indication yesterday that the inoculations at the Waldorf-Astoria had not failed to "take." The waiters made way for each other with a solicitude that sprang from something more than politeness, and the elevator boys became excessively uneasy when their glided cages were uncomfortably crowded.

THE BURDEN OF BONAPARTE.

He Is Suffering From a Name Inflicted by a Father Upon His Son.

From the New York Sun.

"I wasn't born cross-eyed nor club-footed," said the man from Montana, "nor made a vicious bide at the end of a fresh cigar," and things have gone fairly well with me in a business way, but yet there is one thing which never comes up to me that I don't feel like committing murder. My father named me Bonaparte. As a child I was, of course, called Bony, but as soon as old enough to get out into the street the boys shortened that to Bones, and Bones I am to this day. I'm telling you that no man who is Bill or Joe or Tom ever gets up in the world beyond a certain point. He may be known as a good fellow, but your familiarity with him loses him your respect and you undervalue him. Let a man get a nickname after he has conquered fame and it helps him, but people care not helping Jacks and Jims and Petes to congressional honors or governorships. That name of Bones excited ridicule and contempt. I licked fifty different kids for loading it on me, but it stuck. I went to Sunday school and day school as Bones. I went to college and to business as Bones. If my name had been George or Reginald

WELTMERISM

Marks a New Era in the Science of Curing Diseases of All Kinds—The Achievements by This Wonderful Method Have Been So Astounding That It Has Revolutionized the Art to Cure—Medicines a Thing of the Past.

SCIENCE CROWNS PROFESSOR S. A. WELTMER, THE FOUNDER, AS HUMANITY'S GREATEST BENEFACTOR.

TESTED BY 24,000 AFFLICTED AND FOUND INFALLIBLE.

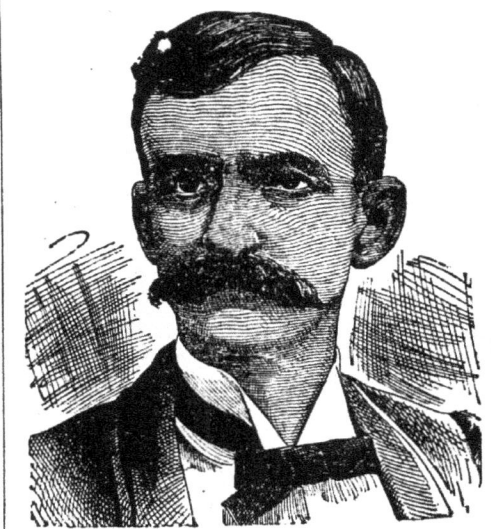

PROF. S. A. WELTMER.

Professor S. A. Weltmer, the great scientist, of Nevada, Mo., has made magnetic healing a positive science. So many cures have been made by this great invisible power that medical men and scientists throughout the civilized world are assured that Weltmerism is destined to attain supreme empire over diseases of all kinds and thereby revolutionize the art of cure. This great science is, indeed, a jeweled weapon, which makes humanity master over its own fate. For, give humanity perfect health, and you give it the key to the gateway of success. Too often has the cure by medicines proven more harmful than the disease. Too often has the surgeon's knife proven dangerous. Weltmerism at last gives to the world a method whereby the constitution is not ruined with strong drugs nor the limbs crippled by the deadly knife, for it dispels all afflictions without the aid of either medicines or the surgeon's knife. Eminent preachers throughout the country have made this boon to humanity the text of their sermons

Weltmer is the greatest curative power of the age.—New York Journal.

The phenomenal cures made by Professor S. A. Weltmer, of Nevada, Mo., have been so astounding as to attract the attention of scientists and physicians throughout the world.—St. Louis Post-Dispatch.

Thousands upon thousands of ailing people have been cured by Professor S. A. Weltmer, the great Nevada, Mo., Magnetic Healer.—Kansas City Star.

Our fellow-townsman, whom we all love and honor for his generosity and kindness, and for making Nevada, Mo., famous by his many noted cures, is deservingly termed the world's greatest benefactor.—Nevada (Mo.) Mail.

Hon. Press Irons, mayor of Nevada, was afflicted with kidney and bladder troubles for ten years and could find no relief in the usual remedies. In one week he was completely restored by Professor Weltmer.

Mr. John S. Small, Colfax, Ill., was deaf in his left ear for seven years; could not hear a watch tick when placed against this ear. Was permanently cured in three days by Professor Weltmer. Mr. L. W. Rains, a wealthy lumberman of Hornbeak, Tenn., suffered constantly with kidney trouble for

kins, Louisburg, Ka with prolapsus an womb, indigestion Tried everything gave up in despair mer, took his treat permanently restore

Prof. Weltmer als ble ability to cure hundreds have bee Mr. G. W. Hightoy a total wreck, live with stomach, live Tried everything w stored by Prof. We

Mrs. Minnie L. was afflicted for 18 other diseases, an to get out of her die at any time. Prof. Weltmer's A gained 6 pounds. for 38 years with troubles. Nothing lieve her. Perma weeks by the Abs ment.

Mrs. M. A. Dev afflicted five year and kidney troubl from medical scien by Absent Treatm

Mrs. M. M. Wa fered with eczema troubles. Douglas any relief. She w by Professor Weltm two months.

Mrs. Jennie L. was for two years of the womb, hea and general debilit skeleton. After ta medicines without Weltmer Absent thirty days she w gained fifteen pou

Professor S. A. ment is, indeed, i and on account o to all classes of p nor condition mak The Weltmer me it can be positive to go to Nevada, will reach and giv they live, no mat

Thousands of p the United States tries who are in various diseases through the powe absent treatment, ed annihilates spa that no matter w what distance the lief from the W writing to Profes vada, Mo., will re trated magazine from men and wo and happiness to information on th

THE WELTME TO

This Noble Profes Fame and Fo

Professor S. A. of the marvelous Weltmerism, will how to cure ever the aid of drugs o one who desires c sion. Anyone who has abundantly number who has and who are in t ing by his method big success in th the method whic Prof. S. A. Welt eminent preacher

Prof. S. A. Welt Dear Brother mail I send you Journal. I than made me happy Magnetic Healing have been havi pleasing results. With best wis

THE WAY TO HEALTH, PROSPERITY, HAPPINESS

The Easy, Inspiring, Practical Weltmer Way
Principles and Practice of

MAGNETIC HEALING, SUGGESTION THERAPY, CHRISTIAN HEALING, MASSAGE

Five Weeks Resident Course

Weltmer Institute
(Established 1897)

Nevada, Missouri

Complete Daily Program

WHAT YOU WILL LEARN

9:00 to 9:30 A.M. HEALING SERVICE

Every day at the Weltmer Institute begins with the Morning Healing Service. In a darkened room, with some people lying on treatment
tables, others relaxing in comfortable chairs, a teacher gives a lesson in relaxation and an inspiring healing lesson for the benefit of
those physically and those only spiritually present.

This is a healing service for the sick of all the world. People
in many lands attune their minds to this group each day and are blessed by the healing thoughts that they feel that they receive. .

The teacher rarely chooses the subject of the lesson beforehand;
usually he comes to the lesson sensitized to the thoughts and the need
of those gathered together there. If one of those physically present h
some certain great need the teacher usually feels and responds to that
need with the necessary lesson. Sometimes the need of one far distant
in the flesh but present in spirit, guides the teacher in his choice of
the subject of the lesson.

So universal is the teaching in the Morning Healing Service, that
everyone who comes physically or only spiritually is blessed according to his ability to receive.

10.00 to 10:30 A. M. PRACTICAL MAGNETIC HEALING

This resident course in Magnetic Healing strikes a new note in
therapeutic instruction. The Weltmer practitioner does not treat disease, he treats the sick and he treats them for the awakening of the
deeper powers of life by which all healing is done. The Weltmer healer
is a true "healer". He is not a doctor, he is not a diagnostician, he
is a healer, by the power of the awakened consciousness of the Kingdom
within.

Weltmer Resident Course (pg 1)
(SHSMO) State Historical Society of Missouri artifact
(Courtesy of the Bushwhacker Museum, Nevada, Mo.)

160

Papa is downtown where he stays most all the time, only when he wants something to eat

Mary Wilson's, Page 2
1903 letter to Lizzie
"Papa is downtown where he stays most all the time, only (comes home) when he wants something to eat."
(Author's collection)

Lester's Mother's Day Card, May 1918 (WWI)
Naval Air Station, La Trinite, France
(Author's collection)

gone! All the same, she would rather a good night's sleep until she hears he has landed... I keep thinking what a different world it will be to us others; when you all come marching home again!

And when you do come marching home,— bring me back the same boy I gave my country,— true, & clean, & gentle, & brave. You need do this for your father & me & Betty & Nora;— & most of all, for the daughter you will give to me one of these days! Dear, I don't know whether you have even met her yet,— but never mind that! Live for her & if God wills, die for her;— but do either with courage,— "with honour & clean mirth!" But I know you will come back to me —

Mother

Lizzie's reply in Mother's Day Card, Page 2, May 1918
Mailed back to Lester at the Naval Air Station, La Trinite, France
(Author's collection)

American Association of United Drugless Physicians

Spokane, Washington,
June 21, 1920.

Dr. S. L. Snyder,
Hoquiam, Wash.

Dear Doctor:

Do you desire to render a greater measure of service? Do you love to help humanity? Are you willing to learn how much you can count in the advancement of National Medical Freedom? Then come to the State and National Convention of United Drugless Physicians at Vancouver, Washington, June 28, 29 and 30th, Elks' Temple.

You can help to save and advance your interest in this and every State in the United States.

There will be work in the convention to engage the mind of each and every one who attends and which will challenge his highest thought.

The character of work to be done will be such that, when completed, it will stand as a monument to the collective thought and efforts of those attending, and will mark it as the most advanced and constructive convention ever held by a like gathering of people in this country.

You will meet delegates from all of the Pacific Coast States who are imbued with a noble purpose to render a still greater measure of service to humanity in co-operation with you.

Come and help to lay the foundation of an organization that will meet every need of every separate and co-ordinate system of natural therapy, as well as the need and welfare of every practitioner of such system; an organization that will meet every wish and will with an open receptive mind and that will function true to the best interests of humanity--Medical Freedom.

We urge that you arrange your affairs so that you may be able to join with us in the FIRST effort to construct the greatest composite Association in the United States for the promotion of natural methods of caring for the public health.

This is a real call--the call of humanity for safer, saner and more rational ways and means of helping those in their hour of affliction.

When you come to Vancouver and experience the spirit of this Convention you will be glad of the opportunity it afforded you. You will want to attend the next one, even though it may cost you a little time, money and inconvenience.

Please accept this letter as a personal invitation, from the Convention Committee, to attend.

Wishing you the best of health and continued success, believe us,

Fraternally,

CONVENTION COMMITTEE

Dr. J. E. Lydon

Chairman.

National Convention, Vancouver, WA
American Association of United Drugless Physicians
(June 21, 1920)
(Author's collection)

164

The American University of Sanipractic

1134 SEVENTEENTH AVENUE
(at E. Union St.)

Dr. S. L. Snyder,
Dear Doctor: Seattle, Wash., July 28, 1920.

Opportunities come and go. They often depart unheeded and return no more. A great opportunity is now at your door.

Dr. Gregory, the greatest author of rational therapy methods and the most successful teacher of Postgraduate Courses, who has gathered so much practical and helpful information since beginning his public lectures ten years ago, is now in Seattle and will conduct a special Postgraduate course beginning August 2nd, 8 p.m., at American University of Sanipractic, corner Seventeenth and East Union.

Dr. Gregory is getting wonderful results by using his combined drugless methods, usually overcoming, with a single treatment, such diseases as appendicitis, angina pectoris, diarrhoea, diphtheria, "flu," pneumonia, scarlet fever, tic-dou-loureux, acute tonsilitis, lumbago and sciatica and other acute diseases.

Dr. Gregory, by use of his special methods, restores to normal in from 3 to 6 treatments, cases of asthma, constipation, cystitis, dysmenorrhea, epitheloma, gonorrhea, hay fever, heart diseases (weakness dilation, regurgitation, etc.), loss of sexual power, etc.

Dr. Gregory has successfully restored to health cases of Bright's disease, diabetes millitis, chronic catarrh, cataracts of the eye, inflammatory rheumatism, syphilis, etc., in from 6 to 30 treatments. Dr. Gregory reduces high blood pressure, from as high as 240 to normal, in from 2 to 3 weeks, and stops hemorrhage from the nose, lungs, stomach, kidneys, uterus, and other parts of the body in a minute's time in most all cases.

How Dr. Gregory obtains these wonderful results will be taught and clearly explained in the Seattle special course of two weeks and this "doctor" is your chance to get this information for a very low tuition.

Dr. Gregory's continued success and the universal satisfaction he has always given, is evidence of the merits of his courses of instruction; and the facts that progressive doctors take his course repeatedly year after year because they, each time, get so much new, helpful matter; and the facts that his recent students are now getting more and better results with three treatments than with ten treatments using former methods, are enough to convince the wise and progressive. The opportunity is yours. May we meet you face to face August 2, 8 p.m., at Sanipractic University, 17th Avenue and East Union Street?

Take cars No. 8 or 10 on Third Avenue.

Fraternally Yours,
AMERICAN UNIVERSITY OF SANIPRACTIC.

The American University of Sanipractic
Dr. Gregory post-graduate course
(July 28, 1920)
(Author's collection)

SELECTED BIBLIOGRAPHY

Books:

Behncke, F.H. *Pioneer Teachers*, originally published 1920, Reprint: Kessinger Publishing, Author's collection.

Brooke, Elisabeth. *Woman Healers: Portraits of Herbalist, Physicians, and Midwives,* Healing Arts Press, Rochester, Vermont,1995.

Campbell, Olivia. *Women in White Coats*, Park Row Books, Toronto, Ontario, Canada, 2022.

Ehrenreich, Barbara/English, Deirdre. W*itches, Midwives & Nurses: A History of Women Healers,* Feminist Press, NY, 2010,

U.S. National Library of Medicine. *Glances and glimpses, or Fifty years social, including twenty years professional life*, Harriot Kezia Hunt, Boston: J.P. Jewett and Co, 1856.

Van Syckle, Edwin. *The River Pioneers: Early Days on Grays Harbor*, Pacific Search Press, Seattle, WA 1982.

Weltmer, Prof. S.A.:

- o *Mystery Revealed,* published 1901, Hudson-Kimberly Publishing Co., Kansas City, Mo.,Stanford University Libraries, digitized, public domain.

- o *Regeneration,* published (copyrighted) 1898, 1900, 1908, Combe Press, St. Joseph, Mo. (Author's collection).

- o *The Healing Hand,* published May 1922-Apr 1925, Weltmer Foundation, Nevada, Mo., digitized, public domain.

- o *How to Succeed,* published 1912, The Weltmer Institute of Suggestive Therapeutics Company, Nevada, Mo., National Archives, digitized, public domain.

Whorton, James C, *Ph.D. Nature Cures: The History of Alternative Medicine in America,* Oxford University Press, NY, 2002.

Articles:

Brophy, Patrick. *Missouri Historical Review;* "Weltmer, Stanhope, and the Rest: Magnetic Healing in Nevada, Missouri," 277, April 1997

166

About the Author

KB Taylor's Grays Harbor family history spans back to the 1880's. She worked as a project-control manager for an aerospace contractor in San Diego and now resides with her husband in Washington State. Historical writing has become her bliss, and with such a colorful lineage, she incorporates them into her books.

Historical fiction by the author:

WILLA Award winner:

- *The Seagirls of the Irene,* Book 1 of the Seagirl's Adventure series. (Children)

WILL ROGERS Medallion Award winners:

- *Hattie's Family: Through the eyes of a Dairymaid* (Western Romance), which features the author's magic-healer grandfather.
- *Forging Through Unknowns: The Seagirls' Alaskan Adventure,* Book 2 of the Seagirl's Adventure series. (Children/YA)

Non-fiction:

- *8138 th Army Unit Hospital Trains, Korean War,* told through firsthand accounts of the author's aunt, a nurse on the hospital trains, and from a medic as they cared for the wounded on their journey from the frontlines.

www.kb-Taylor.com